DON'T BUY TOO MANY
GREEN BANANAS

Living with ALS
(Lou Gehrig's Disease)

Delores M. Warner

D1473742

Lady Peacock Press
Auburn, Washington

DON'T BUY TOO MANY
GREEN BANANAS:
Living with ALS
(Lou Gehrig's Disease)

Delores M. Warner

Dedication

This book is dedicated to my children, Desiree, Sirena, and Derek: my sons-in-law Patrick Sagdahl and Gene Cernilli: my grandchildren, Dustin, Morgan, Erika, Nathaniel, Cole and Tess - all of whom lived, witnessed, and endured our journey during this ordeal.

Acknowledgements

This was not an easy book to write, reliving the experience was emotionally draining. The help and input of my children, Desiree, Sirena, Derek, and friend, Mary North made the challenge easier. They reminded me of incidents that happened which I had not recorded in my journal, so that I could include them in the book.

I would like to acknowledge the expertise of my sister-in-law, Ann Warner for editing, and encouragement, along with my friend, Marjorie Rommel, for their reviews and suggestions on making the story flow more smoothly. I'd also like to acknowledge Sue Sayles for her initial editing of the first draft, and the emails she'd saved during Vern's illness and sent to me after I started the book. They helped fill in events I'd not recorded in my journal.

Thank you to Sonja Zimmer for reviewing the story and giving me recent information on ALS which was so helpful in keeping things accurate and up to date. Also to Mike Webb who kept me posted on new benefits and services that Veterans Affairs offers to veterans and their families, both while Vern was alive, as well as after he'd passed away, keeping that information current. I also appreciate his support during these times.

Thanks to my friend, Claris O'Connor, who is a Master Graphoanalyst, for pointing out typos she found while reviewing the book. Another Master Graphoanalyst, my friend, Winnie Walters, who is a former Whitworth College instructor reviewed the book. Dr. Bob Baugher, a professor at Highline Community College, also reviewed the book.

Last but not least my appreciation to Denise Fuller for her final editing of this book and willingness to take on a first time author, to Ron Engstrom of Desktop Publishing for printing the book, and to David Kelliher of Creative Solutions for the cover design.

All of these people helped make the book what it is today. I can't thank them enough for taking their valuable time to do this for me.

Introduction

Every ninety minutes, someone in the United States is diagnosed with Amyotrophic Lateral Sclerosis (ALS), a disease that affects five out of every one-hundred thousand people worldwide. Only someone who has experienced being told they have ALS can truly know what that is like. It has to be the kind of horrifying news that can only be accepted and acknowledged gradually.

The story you are about to read is how one of the people caught by those odds, LaVerne (Vern) Warner, and his family lived and coped after the diagnosis. Certainly for my husband Vic, Vern's youngest brother, and for me, that news was something we had difficulty fully comprehending for some time.

When Vern graduated from high school, Vic was still in grade school, so the two did not share a close sibling relationship as youngsters, and as adults, their lives went in very different directions.

Vern served in the Army in Germany during the Korean conflict, and it may have been something about this experience that triggered his ALS. It has now been recognized that veterans have a sixty percent higher risk of developing ALS than non-veterans, regardless of service branch or time period served. In fact, the relationship is so strong that Congress recently passed a bill into law that makes ALS a service-related disability.

After returning from Germany, Vern worked in construction and eventually owned his own company which built many stores for Nordstrom's in the Pacific Northwest and Alaska during the pipeline era.

Vic went to college at the University of Washington and then to graduate school at the University of Kansas where he met me, and the two of us married and lived in Boston, Puerto Rico, and finally Cincinnati. That meant our contact with Vern and Delores consisted of brief family visits. However, as the years passed, the four of us became more than people forced into contact by family ties. We became dear friends. And so when Vern received that awful diagnosis, it affected us deeply.

Vic immediately planned a series of visits to Seattle. During one of those visits, we managed to go with Vern and Delores to their favorite restaurant for the last time. We also spent hours listening to Vern tell Warner family stories.

Vern was a great raconteur, and he knew stories from before Vic was born. We eventually thought to record them, so that we now have both the stories as well as a way to hear, once again, Vern's voice. Vern was lucky in that many ALS patients eventually lose their ability to speak, but he never did.

Most patients remain sharp mentally, even as their bodies continue to fail. This was true of Vern. Up to the last, his mind was clear and he was engaged with life, able to talk about his illness and even able to find humor in his condition. That meant our visits together were mostly joyful and those visits left us with memories we treasure.

Vern was the third oldest in his family of five siblings but was the one everybody depended on. He and Delores even took in a friend dying of cancer and cared for him in their home during his last days. Vern was an executor for the estates of a number of friends and family, and he was the person we called whenever we were in need of his unique blend of wisdom--a practical knowledge of how most things worked tempered by common sense. He was generous to a fault and always more than willing to share his expertise and his time. His neighbors knew him as someone they could rely on to help them whenever they needed it so it was no surprise to us that these neighbors rallied round after Vern's diagnosis.

Delores continues to live on the two and a half acres that she and Vern bought forty-eight years ago in a house she designed and he built. They raised three children -- Desiree, Sirena, and Derek.

Unwilling to give up his agrarian roots, as well as wanting to expand his children's experiences, Vern stocked their property, as well as leasing 20 acres adjoining their property, with a variety of animals. Vic, during his years at the University, ate better because Vern raised pigs, cattle, and sheep. When they were butchered, he shared the meat with the entire family, charging only his direct costs, making a gift of his time and effort.

Although he stopped raising pigs, cattle, and sheep a number of years ago, Vern and Delores continued to keep horses, goats, chickens, and even peafowl. Vern delighted in sharing his mini-farm with the neighborhood children, who were equally delighted to discover where eggs come from.

Vern was a problem solver and, for him, that was how he faced this disease -- figuring out, with Delores's help, how to deal with many of the physical obstacles they had to face.

ALS starts with the degeneration of the nerve cells which enervate the muscles responsible for voluntary movement. Without the nerves doing their job, these muscles waste away (atrophy). Gradually, the patient with ALS becomes paralyzed, unable to walk, to move their arms, to talk, to breathe. The end result of this progressive muscle weakness, if the patient doesn't die of pneumonia or related illnesses, is a condition called Locked In Syndrome -- a state where patients can't move or speak, but their minds remain clear.

ALS patients do not lose their five senses and rarely does the disease affect bowel or bladder function. Once diagnosed, most patients have a life expectancy between two to five years and although there are cases where the disease progression seems to "burn out", only twenty-five percent of patients survive beyond five years.

There are still many unanswered questions about what causes ALS. A genetic component has been identified but it appears to be responsible for only ten percent of cases. The other ninety percent of cases are classified as sporadic and appear to arise spontaneously. No clear risk factors or direct causes of the disease have been established, and no two patients will experience the same progression of symptoms.

After Vern's diagnosis, he continued, with Delores's help, to live as fully as possible. The two of them had the gift of making casual strangers into life-long friends and so they had many friends to share the road they were forced to travel. Vern was no saint, as you will discover as you read this book, but he (and Delores) faced his fate with a strength and grace that has been an inspiration to all of us who witnessed it. None of us, however, walked every inch of that road as Delores did.

Through this book, which is based on the journals and emails she wrote during that time, she shares the entire journey with us.

Ann M. Warner

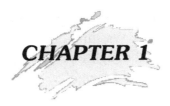

CHAPTER 1

At the sound of Vern's footsteps coming down the hallway after his appointment with the first neurologist, I turned from preparing a snack for our lunch and asked, "Well, what did she say?"

"She said I have Lou Gehrig's Disease."

His response stunned me. All I could say was, "That's not good."

He continued, "She wants me to go to the University of Washington Medical Center (UWMC) for confirmation. But, she said she's sure that it is ALS."

"I hope she's wrong!" I knew if the neurologist was right, it was a death sentence. That was all either of us knew about amyotrophic lateral sclerosis (ALS) also known as Lou Gehrig's Disease. It was a total shock to us. The date was January 20, 2009.

Vern had always been the strong one, the born leader, independent and self sufficient, while I played a more supportive role in the family, more easy going, relaxed, sympathetic and patient.

Many times I had to go deep within myself to gather up strength I never knew I had because I wanted to help this man whom I loved, in order to help him go through this ordeal as comfortably as possible.

As a youngster, one of Vern's jobs was breaking horses. He had those natural cowboy traits and loved to watch western movies. He was a cowboy at heart, strong willed, decisive, and a US army veteran. Before moving into our present home, we lived in a mobile home for several years. But, we both wanted more space and a small acreage to raise our family. We purchased two and a half acres in the Auburn,/Federal Way, Washington area. He bought a Shetland pony for our six year old daughter, Desiree. That was the start of our little mini-farm. Second daughter, Sirena, was born the night we moved to this property.

How was he going to face this disease if it was confirmed to be ALS?

Going back to December 15, 2008, while helping a friend with frozen water pipes Vern had a nasty fall on the icy sidewalk. He tore his groin muscles and his right hamstring. He had bruises on his right buttocks, in his groin area, and on his right leg, front and back to his knee. In the days that followed, as one bruise would clear up another would emerge.

For two weeks he managed to get around using a crutch but was unable to get to his primary physician's office. We had to reschedule his dentist appointment. Since he also couldn't get dressed, he wore pajamas, and as I ironed a pair one morning, I jokingly said to him I had my own handsome Hugh Hefner lounging around, but with fewer adoring female fans hanging all over him.

Once he was able to get up and around, we both noticed he was losing more and more strength in his arms and hands. We thought possibly it was his statin medication, so he went off it for several weeks, but he only continued to get weaker.

The first part of January, during his recuperation, he visited his primary physician several times trying to get to the bottom of his increasing weakness. Mid-January, his doctor referred him to a neurologist in Auburn, Washington

He was sitting in the exam room at the neurologist's office when in walked the petite Asian doctor. She asked him to strip to his waist. She pulled up her stool and stared at his bare chest. She could see the nerves twitching in his arms and body. She ordered magnetic resonance imaging (MRI) and electromyography (EMG) tests, a spinal tap, and blood and urine tests.

The neurologist quizzed him, "Surely you must have suspected ALS?"

He answered, "I've never known anyone that had it. I know nothing about it except people die from it, like Lou Gehrig. That's what I know about it."

I began searching my memory to locate the point in time when he first noticed a considerable decline in his muscle strength.

I remembered that for the past few years, Vern had scared me while driving the car and pickup. He'd always been an excellent driver, so I should have known at the time something was wrong. It sometimes seemed as if he didn't have complete control of the car.

Derek is in his forties, single and is the youngest of our three children. He owns his own home and lives about two miles from our home. Derek spent a lot of time with us. Derek and I had talked about Vern's driving in a joking manner, and we teased him, never realizing something was seriously wrong. Derek has a great sense of humor (I like to think he got that from me) but, Vern would joke back and we'd all have a good laugh.

One day we picked up our grandchildren from school, and Vern couldn't turn the key in the ignition. Ten year old Nathaniel had to do it for him. He decided then it was time for him to stop driving.

I also remembered that in early 2008 he noticed he could no longer pull the cords to start either his chain saw or the lawn mower. Also, he noticed that other things he was used to doing with no problem were now difficult or impossible. He offered to open a jar of juice one morning and couldn't. He had difficulty reaching into the cupboard for a cup. He thought it was his age catching up with him. He was 74 at the time.

Wanting to learn more about the disease I checked the Internet.

I discovered that ALS is a progressive and usually fatal disorder which affects the nerve cells that control voluntary movement. As the nerve cells in the brain and spinal cord gradually degenerate they cause the muscles under their control to weaken and waste away.

The email I sent to our daughters, Desiree and Sirena said,

> I just want you girls to know that if it turns out to be ALS, I will face it as a challenge to take care of your dad. And I'm up to the challenge. I just hate for him to have to go through what he faces down the road. I may get emotional from time to time but please bear with me as you both know that is my personality. Sorry, but that is the way I am. I know I have a lot of support so I'm not feeling sorry for me as I know I can handle it. I just feel bad for him. I will keep my chin up and learn as much as I can about what I need to do to help him.
>
> Love, Mom

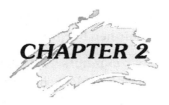

CHAPTER 2

February 2009

The morning of February 26th, Vern went out to do the chores. He couldn't get the key in the lock to unlock the gate going into the pasture. He came back to the house with moist eyes. I thought there might be a tear about to fall. "I can't do the chores any more. I can't even unlock the damn gate."

Since his fall the previous December, I had offered to do them many times, but he was determined he was going to do them. He loved being with his animals, but that morning brought the realization he couldn't do that any longer.

Sirena always idealized her father, and he absolutely adored her. He loved Desiree and Derek as well, but he and Sirena just had a special relationship. They were alike in many ways, both were goal-oriented, self confident, and liked to delegate work; both made good bosses. Sirena is more emotional and demonstrative than her father, and she has a wonderful bubbly personality that people love to be around. On March 4th, Sirena drove us to the UWMC for our consultation with the MDA/ALS neurologist. Vern had great difficulty taking his sweater off, and Sirena helped him with that.

The tests took all day. This second neurologist asked Vern to get an additional MRI of the thorax area and L-spine to give her a complete MRI of his spine. She also did a thorough neurological examination.

It was a long day for Vern and he was exhausted. Still, on the way home from the medical center, Vern asked Sirena if she'd like to pick up dinner for her family. We'd pay for it, since she had spent the whole day with us. We stopped at our favorite Mom and

Pop restaurant, Yummy Teriyaki. When the order was ready, Vern couldn't get out of the chair he'd been sitting in.

Sirena, an emergency room nurse, lifts patients at the hospital all day and she thought she could help him out of the chair by herself. She was stunned that he had no strength to help her. The owner of the restaurant had to help us get him out of the chair and back to the car. This would be one of the indelible memories of Vern's decline.

Our other daughter, Desiree, who is six years older than Sirena, lives in New York. She is a talented actress and went to New York to study acting at the age of twenty-one, taking that opportunity to get away from the strained relationship she had with her dad. Vern was a person who liked to control those around him and was possessive of his family. While the rest of us tolerated that, Desiree was anxious to get away from what she thought of as the "control freak."

Vern was a pusher, and a take charge person, and Desiree didn't like being pushed into doing things at his immediate request. She is more laidback and likes to do things in her own time. She is compassionate, something that Vern was not, and she likes the arts, something her dad didn't understand.

Desiree had planned on coming to visit with her family during the summer months when their children were on vacation. Sirena called them that evening and told them, "If you want your kids to have positive memories of their grandfather, you need to come during spring break."

Their family did come to visit before the final consultation date with the second neurologist, which was at the UWMC. Desiree had met her husband when she first went to New York where they both were working at a theater. They now had two young children, Cole and Tess.

There was a certain amount of freedom in not knowing the true diagnosis of ALS at that point. Vern took Cole and Tess out to help feed the animals, and they thought it was a lot of fun, throwing the hay to the horses, tossing the feed for the peafowl and chickens, and giving grain to the goats and horses. In reality it was helping Vern as he couldn't lift his arms high enough to do those things. We had a wonderful visit.

Three weeks after our initial appointment at the UWMC, we returned. The neurologist confirmed the diagnosis was ALS. Sirena and I couldn't hold back the tears. The doctor offered us a box of tissues.

Vern asked the neurologist, "What do we do from here? Give it to me straight. I want to know what to expect down the road. Don't hold anything back."

"The disease paralyzes the voluntary muscles, but you will remain alert and be able to think clearly," the doctor said. "Your five senses will be unaffected, and some patients maintain control over their bowels and bladder. You will gradually become completely paralyzed and will only able to move your eyes. Eventually you may have difficulty talking. So far there is no known cure. There is a medication, Rilutek, that has proven to stabilize it for approximately three months at the stage it is now, but the disease will eventually continue to worsen."

"If it isn't going to cure the disease, then why prolong the end?" Vern asked her.

"Because it may give you an added three months, maybe a little more, to enjoy life at the stage you are in now."

Vern refused the medication. It was expensive, and most people refuse it because they can't afford it, but even knowing the medication would be paid for by the VA , Vern still said "No."

As we were leaving the neurologist's office, she remembered that one of the representatives from the ALS Association was at the hospital in her unit. She asked if we'd like to meet her. When we said we would, she had her come in and tell us a little about what the Association does for the ALS patients. She gave us a contact number for the Evergreen Chapter of ALS in Kent, Washington, if we needed help with anything.

Vern didn't say much on the way home. I had to keep looking out the car window so he wouldn't see the tears falling down my cheeks. Although I'm sure he saw me wiping them away. He disliked tears and emotions, but the tears continued to fall. It was a difficult drive home.

When Derek took Vern to his primary care physician following the confirmation of his ALS diagnosis, his doctor pointed out that he'd probably had the disease for five to six years, though we didn't know it until the fall he took in December put the disease into high gear.

"Any sort of trauma, an auto accident, a divorce, and in your case, your fall in December, will escalate the disease," the doctor told him. The only hopeful thing he had to say was that he had another patient with ALS who was diagnosed at age 20 and was now 30.

Vern felt a little more optimistic after that, but I was beginning to understand how devastating it was going to be for this man who had always been so active all his life. A hard worker, a man who had at one time owned his own commercial construction business, and now had a little mini farm. A man people came to when they needed help.

Vern also served as executor for a number of friends and family members, and was always willing to help others in need of his expertise, with no expectation of anything in return. He now faced a future of complete dependency on others. It was a fact he hated. He was used to being in charge of everyone and everything. How was he going to cope?

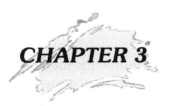

CHAPTER 3

The night after the diagnosis was confirmed, neither of us slept much, thinking about what was in store for us. I found myself wiping tears away before falling asleep. The next morning as we sat having coffee in our pajamas Vern said, "Please do not put me in a nursing home."

"I would never put you in a nursing home. We'll face this challenge together and I'll always be here for you. I promise I will take care of you until the end." And I broke down crying.

Vern did as well. It was only the second time I'd seen him cry in the fifty six years we'd been married. The other time was when his older brother Lloyd was killed in a car accident. They had been very close, as they worked in the construction business together. I'm not sure he ever got over the loss of his brother.

I knew why Vern was asking me not to put him in a nursing home. Both of us had had bad experiences with our mothers in nursing homes. His mother was in one for two years in a coma before she passed away. It was awful. It smelled bad, and people lay calling for help. We visited often, and each time we did, we found her lying in her own waste and had a hard time getting an aide to come clean her up.

My mother had better care in a different nursing home and I visited almost every day. They were good to her, but suddenly she was unresponsive to my being there. I asked what medication she was on, and the staff refused to tell me. I called her doctor and he said he had never seen her in the condition I described to him, so I asked him when the last time he saw her was. He checked his records and it had been five weeks. I gave him a piece of my mind and told him if he didn't have time to check on her I'd get another doctor.

The next day when I visited my mother the charge nurse asked me what I had said to the doctor, because he was really furious with me about my phone call. I was told he changed her medications.

A few months later when she was moved to another wing of the nursing home, one of the nurses accidentally gave her another patient's medicine and I was called to take her to the hospital as there wasn't an ambulance available at the time. She lived only a few weeks more, but passed away after that episode because of the nurse's error.

I had worked six years for a doctor who had several nursing home patients. When they were brought into the office, they were like zombies from being over medicated; some had ulcers from sitting in their own urine. Some complained that in the nursing home their call lights were ignored. Remembering all these experiences, I knew I could never put Vern into a nursing home, but I also knew I would have to have help to care for him. Our daughter, Sirena, lives across town and could help. I knew, in particular, I could count on Derek to come when I needed him. Our daughter in New York, Desiree, even though she was thousands of miles away, was a great moral support with phone calls.

Derek is happy with his life, gets along well with others, but his relationship with his father was somewhat difficult, maybe because they were at opposite ends of the personality spectrum. They worked together on many projects, but when they did, Vern always pointed out what Derek did wrong, rather than complimenting him when he did something right. It wasn't in Vern's nature to give compliments. In fact, it was true of our relationship as well, and he often made me feel stupid.

Derek eventually decided, "Dad wasn't necessarily picking on me, but as a kid I thought he was." Over the years, Derek and I tried to please Vern, and we did point out to him when he was wrong about something, but it was a losing battle. Vern would never admit he was wrong, and he could never say "I'm sorry."

On the other hand, Vern's critical nature and lack of tolerance for mistakes were what made him a commercial building contractor in demand. People knew he was a perfectionist in his work. Vern's personalized license plate at that time said it all: DBOSS. As did his favorite quote: "Better them pissed off than me." If Vern was upset about something, or someone, you knew it, he let you know he was angry.

One day one of his employees went home and told his wife that his butt felt like hamburger. When she asked him why, he answered, "Because Vern has been chewing on it all day." Vern was inflexible and somewhat short tempered. He had no patience.

The possibility that Vern had ALS was first raised on January 20, 2009. By March 10th, he could no longer brush his teeth, and couldn't reach up to comb his hair. He needed help to put on his shirts and button them up. He struggled with pulling up his pants. Derek came by each morning to help me get Vern dressed and ready for the day.

Vern was very particular about his hair, even though at this stage of his life he didn't have much left. It had to be done just the way he'd combed it all his life. One day as Derek was combing his hair, Vern was watching in the mirror to make sure it was done to his satisfaction. It wasn't, and Vern, irritated, told Derek to redo it, "and push up that wave."

Derek tried doing it the way Vern wanted it, each of them getting upset with the other. Finally, Derek put the comb down on the bathroom counter and said, "Wear a damn hat!" And walked out of the room It was the only time he ever lost patience with his dad after the ALS diagnosis.

Only Sirena's ten year old son, Nathaniel, or I could satisfy Vern with the way we combed his hair. Vern started referring to Nathaniel as "The Little Man," because if Nathaniel was here and I was busy doing something else, Nathaniel would step in and put Vern's socks on him and comb his Papa's hair.

In fact Nathaniel had a better way of putting Vern's socks on him than I did. Vern had him show me how he would toss the sock out in front of Vern's foot and pull it on. I had been treating the socks like panty hose and scrunching them up and then pulling. The Little Man's way was much better.

At first Vern didn't have a lot of pain but as the disease progressed so did the pain. And what he could do one week, three weeks later he couldn't do. It seemed like every three weeks he'd lose an ability. Eventually it was each week he'd lose another ability.

He still looked great, though, a handsome man even at the age of seventy-five! And as long as he was sitting in his chair, he appeared to be fine. He had a good attitude about his condition. He would tell people. "I'm glad that it is me and not one of my kids or grandchildren."

I tried to keep him cheerful, so while he stood in the shower and I soaped him down I sang the Hokey Pokey song, changing the lyrics somewhat.

Put your left foot up,

Your left foot down,

Your left foot in,

And shake it all about,

You do the hokey pokey

And turn yourself around

Now put your right arm in

Your right arm out

Right arm in

Then you shake it all about

And then you do the Hokey Pokey

Turn yourself around,

That's what it is all about.

Although Vern had lost control of his arms and hands, he was able to turn around so that I was able to scrub him down. I don't have a very good singing voice, and he always managed to chuckle as I'd start to sing.

These were things that others didn't see because when they visited he was sitting in his chair clean, shaved and dressed, and handsome as ever. They had no idea the struggle he went through letting me do those things for him. Sometimes he'd get tired of me wanting to get every little whisker cut and he'd tell me to just leave it. He had always taken such pride in his appearance and I didn't want that to change.

Eating was becoming difficult for him. As his strength declined he was no longer able to eat at the table. Instead I placed his plate on a serving tray on a low stool. Bending over, he was then able to lift the fork the short distance to his mouth. It was still frustrating for him, as the eating utensils would often turn in his hand.

An occupational therapist eventually brought us a special spoon and fork with a large handle, thinking that would help. She also brought a thing to clip on the side of his plate to help him get the food onto the spoon or fork. These things felt clumsy to him, although they may work well for others. She'd never had an ALS patient before, so it was a new experience for her as well as us.

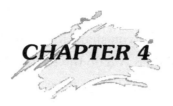

CHAPTER 4

Shortly before Vern was diagnosed, a bill was passed by Congress designating ALS as a military-related disability. This meant that Vern, who had been in the army in the 1950's, was now eligible to receive both care and a disability check from the Veteran's Administration. After we learned of this from a friend of Derek's, I called the Benefits Division, and I was interviewed about Vern and was sent the necessary paperwork to fill out.

About that time a recent acquaintance of ours had come to visit Vern and when Vern mentioned to her that I had contacted the veterans she said, "I have a good friend who works with Disabled Veterans in Seattle. I'll contact him if you'd like or you can contact him yourself."

She gave me his name and phone number, and I called him the next day. He set up an appointment with us and came out and helped me fill out the paperwork. I don't know how I would have ever gotten through it without the help of Mike Webb. He was pleasant, compassionate, helpful and most encouraging. He was a life saver. We are very grateful for all he did for us and the time he spent with us. While Mike was here we had our tearful moments, yes, including Vern--the man who never showed emotions. We all knew it was a dim future we were facing. This was the first case of ALS that Mike had worked with, so we learned a lot together about how the Veteran's Administration would handle this case.

"I'll put on the forms that this needs to be expedited because of Vern's age and it being ALS." Mike said.

Mike made himself available anytime we needed him. Despite our troubles, we were finding all sorts of help in unexpected ways.

Mike was one of those.

As Vern became more and more disabled he also became more and more frustrated with his condition, and on March 11, 2009 he told me to call the Evergreen Chapter of ALS and see if there was something they could do to ease our situation. I was surprised by his request because he was a man who never asked for help. That being so unlike him, I knew he was concerned about his fast ALS progression.

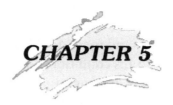

CHAPTER 5

B y April Vern was unable to go outside without help. But each day that he could still get out of bed on his own we felt blessed.

When I showered him in the mornings, I began having difficulty drying him, as he couldn't stand long enough for me to do it. I mentioned this to the occupational therapist, Cathy Barton, and she suggested using a terry-cloth bathrobe instead of a towel. I happened to have a terry cloth robe and I tried it. When I helped him out of the shower, I put the robe on him, then I helped him lie down on the bed, and I'd take a towel and dry his legs and feet. When I'd pull him up in a sitting position and take the robe off he was dry. The "bathrobe trick" as we called it was wonderful and helped a lot.

Getting his shirt and clothes on was a struggle for both of us, but we made it work. In the middle of April I was dressing him and he said, "Somebody sure is mad at me to give me, this disease where I can't even button my shirt." Later in the day he said to Derek, after Derek had gone out and fed the animals, that someone sure was mad at him, because now he couldn't even go out and do the chores.

Vern could shuffle his way to the bed, but by this time he could no longer lift his legs to get into bed by himself. I would help him sit on the edge of the bed, put my arm at his back while also picking his legs up. Once I got his legs on the bed I'd lay him down and cover him up, just like I did our children when they were little.

Our morning cup of coffee together in our pajamas went by the wayside. No time for that. Taking him to the bathroom, bathing him, brushing his teeth, combing his hair, just getting him ready for the day took time.

In early April Vern's brother, Vic, Vic's wife Ann, and son, Eric, came to visit from Cincinnati. We also had company from out of town, and that seemed to lift Vern's spirits. It helped to get his mind off of the disease and got him talking about other things.

I had contacted Vern's good friend George, by mail and told him about Vern's diagnosis. I knew Vern would never tell George because he himself hadn't gotten over the shock yet. When George came to visit, Vern struggled to get out of his chair. Tears rolled down Vern's cheeks and once he composed himself he said "My wife told you, didn't she?" Showing his emotions like that was embarrassing and most difficult for him.

George said, "She wrote me a note." They hugged each other. I poured them coffee and they visited for a long time. .

When Vern did drink something, it took both of his hands to hold a cup or glass, and he had to use a straw as he didn't have the strength or control to drink out of a cup or glass.

Vern found he catnapped more and more. One time he said to me, "I should stay awake more. Once I go to sleep that final time I'll have a lot of time to sleep then, but not now. I should be doing something besides sleeping."

It was so hard on him to not be active. He would look out the windows or the sliding glass door and see things that needed to be done and get upset because he could no longer take care of those things.

The neighborhood children made him a huge "Get Well" poster and brought it to him. He always let them go in the pasture, and watched as the animals and children played together. They adored him, and lovingly called him "Mr. Farmer". He enjoyed sharing his mini farm with the children, teaching them about farm life.

One thing he taught them was about the chickens, that they

only lay one egg a day, that the white chickens laid white eggs and the brown chickens laid brown eggs. He let them gather the eggs. They didn't realize the severity of his disease and really thought he would get well.

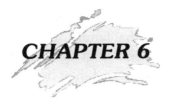

CHAPTER 6

As 2009 turned into 2010, I continued to read everything I could get my hands on about ALS to prepare myself for what was to come. I learned that after a person is diagnosed with ALS, life expectancy is usually two to five years. The cause is unknown, but there are studies that point to the possibility that some cases are hereditary. However, ninety percent have no family history. Risk factors may include tobacco use, poor diet, or exposure to toxins, but no clear cause has been established. Also I learned that every ninety minutes someone is diagnosed with ALS, and every ninety minutes someone with ALS dies.

As I was heading out to do the chores one afternoon Vern asked, "Can I go with you? I really miss being outside and being with the animals. You can hold my arm as I walk out there with you."

I agreed, thinking the outing would be good for him. I went to the shed to get the chicken feed, and when I stepped out I saw him lying on the ground. I had a hard time picking him up.

Another time he fell trying to reach the hummingbird feeder. A neighbor happened to be coming by, and lifted him.

One day our granddaughter, Erika, was mowing the front lawn while Vern was talking to our neighbor Eric, and he just fell to the ground. The two of them had to lift him up.

The time that really embarrassed Vern was when I was mowing the front pasture and he was watching me from the front yard and fell. One of our neighbor ladies who doesn't speak English saw him and tried to pick him up, but couldn't. She had to get another neighbor to help.

The neighbor, who couldn't speak English, had tears running down her cheeks. When that family moved into our neighborhood they were having problems with their heating system and Vern helped them. Later he also fixed their hot tub, their stove and their garage door opener.

I was talking to the owner of the house one day and he said that when they decided to move to America from India, his friends told him, "The Americans don't care about you. They only care about themselves." He went on to say, "After I met Vern and he helped me with the house so much, I told my friends in India, "I met a family in America who cares."

The neighbors all loved Vern. He and our son Derek were always willing to help them with any problems they had. They all became our friends. The support system we had from family and friends like these was unbelievable. In the past Vern had always been Johnny-on-the-spot when it came to helping others, and now we were being repaid many times over.

I never had to call twice about needing help with him. People rallied around when we needed help, many times without our ever asking. Like when the young neighbor boy and his dad came and mowed our lawns. Vern always kept a beautiful well-manicured lawn, so when it needed mowing the neighbors volunteered.

Our grandchildren, Morgan, Erika, and Nathaniel were wonderful help with maintaining the yard. Erika would mow the front pasture, Nathaniel would clean the barn, and Morgan would mow and edge the lawns. If I hadn't already groomed the horses, they would do that, and if Sirena wasn't working at the hospital she would help as well.

May 1, 2009 Sirena and I were brushing the horses. The sun was out, and it was just a beautiful day. We were enjoying what we were doing, she combing one horse and I the other, chatting away. Suddenly, it hit me why the two of us were there together instead of Vern and me. It was times like this where what we were facing would hit me with full force. Most of the time I was so busy doing all I needed to do to take care of Vern, I really didn't have time to dwell on what was yet to come.

My friend, Marjorie, said it best, "Keeping busy is a good veil for sorrow, fear, frustration and loss." Her husband also has medical problems so she knows firsthand.

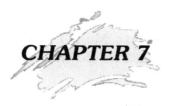

CHAPTER 7

I usually turned the covers down before Vern's bedtime. One evening as I was helping him into bed, he said, "Thank you for turning the bed down for me and tucking me in at night."

I told him, "It's just like the service on a cruise ship, Vern, with a few extra benefits. I never had a cabin steward tuck me in bed or give me a kiss goodnight."

Vern developed a nasty cold in mid-April and it hit him especially hard because of his ALS. He ended up having to have cough syrup, an antibiotic and steroid medication prescribed. The x-rays showed he had a lot of phlegm in his lungs that he had difficulty coughing up as those nerves and muscles were wasting away. That cold lasted him into the second week of May, and created a lot of difficulty breathing .

Vern always raised a beautiful garden and shared his produce with others. Since he couldn't do it after the disease began to take hold, our son-in-law, Pat, rototilled the garden area and planted it for him. Pat, Nathaniel, and sometimes Morgan, kept it weeded. Vern enjoyed watching it grow from inside the house. We all shared the bounty.

One day Pat and Morgan came over to work in the garden. I had given Vern his shower, but I hadn't combed his hair yet. He decided to kneel down for me to do it. When I finished, he couldn't get up. He was embarrassed that Pat and Morgan had witnessed this, and he wiped away tears. I started to cry too, and then Morgan started crying. According to Morgan, "It was 'melt-down' time.."

In May a rotten tree in the woods behind our property fell on our fence. That fence bordered our back pasture. Pat and Derek, who'd just had back surgery, took care of it. As they worked Vern watched, then turned to me and said, "It is so much easier to give than to receive."

I told him, "Over the years you have done so much for others. Now it's your turn to receive."

After the active life Vern had lived, I never imagined that Vern would suffer a gradual decline in health in such a devastating way. It was hard to watch him wither away. If the weather was nice and the sun was shining he did better. On rainy, chilly, or overcast days, he would sleep a lot and go to bed early.

Around the middle of May 2009 Derek noticed that his dad was wiping tears from his eyes for a couple of days. "I think he is going through a bit of depression, Mom," he said to me.

Vern was suffering from a cold again and was having trouble breathing. He was coughing and looking very pale. I'm sure that did depress him. I was worried, and wanted him to contact his doctor for more medication for his cold. He refused. It was as if this time he was giving up rather than wanting to get better. Consequently this cold lasted even longer than the cold he'd had earlier, and he was getting weaker on top of it. It really concerned me.

After his diagnosis, Vern and I both knew we needed to get our financial affairs in order. He had always taken care of the finances, except for my paying the bills. I had no idea how he had invested our money. When I'd wanted to get involved he would push me away. He was always in control.

After a while I decided to let him do whatever he wanted, and not worry about it. But now I needed to know. I had to be involved. When he decided to show me his books where he kept his financial books, they were done in code. Vern's own made up code. The last three months while he was still ambulatory, he tried to show me how to decipher his code. He made me nervous as he stood over my shoulder and urged me to figure it out for myself.

"Why did you do these books in code, Vern?" I asked him one day when he wanted me to record the financial statements as they came in.

"Because it isn't anyone's business if they happen to pick up these records and try to figure them out." I guess that included me. I never got into his desk drawers so had no idea where he kept things or what he kept in them until after he died.

The last time we worked on his books together I still wasn't able to figure out where he got certain figures. He yelled, "I'll never live long enough to show you how to figure it out." He was right. It was after he passed away and I had time to myself without him hovering over me that I figured out his code.

He had other concerns as well. He was scheduled to be the executor for three people's trusts, a responsibility he had to turn back, as he knew he wouldn't live much longer.

We also went to see our trust attorney and updated our own trust. That was an advantage we had; knowing how short the time was, we had time to get our house in order.

Sister-in-law Ann (she's really more like a true sister to me) sent me a book "Home With God" by Neale Donald Walsch. I enjoyed reading it. It mentioned something I've heard many times -- that we all come to earth with a purpose, and once we've completed our purpose, we die.

I have always felt my purpose in life was to help others in any way I can. And it was time for me to help Vern. I was happy to be able to take care of him. I never felt it was a burden. Yet I have to admit there were many mornings when I'd get out of bed and pray for patience just to get through the day. He was never the easiest person to live with. He was often demanding and impatient even before he had ALS.

On June 8, 2009 we received a letter from the Veteran's Administration saying they would schedule an appointment for Vern to take a physical to see what his Range of Motion capabilities were. For the appointment, I made a list of the things he could no longer do and a list of things he had difficulty doing as of June 1, 2009.

Things Vern can No Longer Do:

Drive a vehicle

Walk more than a block (he used to walk 4-6 miles a day)

Mow or edge the lawn

Use the chain saw

Dress himself

Help with the laundry

Comb or shampoo his hair

Fix a plate of food for himself

Cut the food on his plate

Pull his pants up past his buttocks

Cut his own toenails

Vacuum or mop the floors

Hang his clothes up or hang a towel on the towel bar

Put dirty clothes in the hamper

Lie down in bed by himself

Cover himself up in bed

Kneel down without falling over (he is much like a small baby learning to sit up: when he tries to get back up he has no control or strength in his arms to help himself)

De-worm the horses or brush and comb them.

Reach in the cupboards to get anything

Pour himself a cup of coffee

Fill his pill boxes

Raise his arms to wave back at people passing by.

Things He Has Difficulty Doing as of June 2009

He can't reach up past his waist to put soap on his body while showering

He has difficulty eating. He has little control of his hands. The food falls off his eating utensils .

Write -- even to sign his name

All personal hygiene is hard for him to do

Roll over in bed

Put his glasses on to read -- he takes his glasses rests his arm on something. and then leans down to his glasses and tries to put them on.

He gets exhausted when walking only a block. He used to walk 2-4 miles a day for exercise.

I took these lists with us when he had his physical for his Range of Motion tests.

On June 11, 2009, we received word from Veteran's Affairs stating they had evaluated both the ALS specialist's and the neurologist's reports and they were rating him 80% disabled. This was even before he'd had the tests done at the VA, - - it had been such a fast decline in the six months since January when the neurologist first suspected ALS. Now, when a veteran is diagnosed with ALS they are automatically rated 100 percent disabled, because they deteriorate so fast.

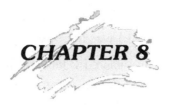

CHAPTER 8

As Vern adjusted to his limitations, we, as his caregivers, had to make major adjustments also. More of my time was now spent taking care of Vern's needs and less on housekeeping, and cooking. And there was no time at all for recreational activities.

One day I'd had enough of his bad humor and I told him, "Vern, you are being grumpy with me."

His response was, "Well, I get impatient, even with myself." That was his way of apologizing. He could never say "I'm sorry"

On June 25, 2009, we had our appointment with the VA doctor who did the Range of Motion test. When he finished he said we would probably get a report in three months. Three months! That seemed like a very long time to have to wait when the patient was declining so rapidly, and the caregiver needed help.

By this time, I had to cut Vern's food up for him. He then struggled to get food in his mouth. Our friend, Inge, came to visit, and I served pie and ice cream but Vern couldn't feed himself. I fed it to him. Afterward Inge said, "I see why he doesn't like to go to restaurants anymore."

Another day he asked Inge to push the button on his lift chair because he didn't have enough control of his hands anymore, and she told me later, "I was shocked that he couldn't use his fingers." He also asked her to move his finger one day because he couldn't and she told me, "I didn't realize how fast he was going downhill."

Several times he told me, "You are the only thing that stands between me and a nursing home now." Taking care of Vern was my priority, and I promised him I'd do it until the end. I had no intention of changing my mind. I wanted to make sure he had the best of care, and I thought I was the one to provide it.

By the first of July he insisted I get a house cleaning service to come help take care of the house. I argued with him about it for a few days as I thought it would be too expensive. He convinced me by saying, "You can't keep the house as clean as we like it and take care of me, so you need help with the house." I gave in. He was right.

We got a bid from a cleaning service. It was expensive but he had me sign up for it. It was one of the best things we did because we ended up with a wonderful house-cleaner, Mary North. She not only cleaned our house well, she became a good friend. While she was at our house, I could even be gone for a few minutes and if Vern needed something, she would get it for him. She remains a good friend to this day. I love her. And so did Vern.

We also hired a young man to come trim the rhododendron bushes, shrubs and ivy, all things Vern and Derek used to do, and I called a window cleaning company to clean the windows. Thus ALS ended up costing us in numerous ways.

At the end of July, Vern's primary care physician arranged for a home nursing care agency to come and evaluate Vern to see which of their services he needed. A physical therapist came first and worked with Vern for one and a half hours. After he left, Vern decided he didn't want him to come back. The next day they sent a nurse out. Vern didn't like her, and asked me to cancel her, but she talked him into having the physical therapist come back. For a time, there were people coming in and out several times a week. In my journal I have written, "Yikes!!" It was starting to get to me.

I felt the physical therapist was exercising Vern to an extreme. I could see the stretching exercises on his arms were hurting him. He would grimace, but he seldom asked the therapist to stop, so I asked him to stop going so far.

"I have to do that in order for him to rebuild his muscles and strength," he said.

"You don't understand. He has ALS, and he will never regain his strength and muscles, and you are hurting him by pulling on his arms." I don't think he ever understood the pain caused by abnormal joint mobility or cramps that are a part of the dreadful ALS.

"He is the first ALS patient I have ever had, but I think he needs to do this to build his strength. He needs to stretch these muscles," he answered me. Many of the educated professionals who took care of Vern seemed to know little if anything about this disease.

Vern wouldn't do the exercises with me that the physical therapist had assigned, and he never slept well the night after the therapist worked with him. The following day his muscles would hurt, and he would be miserable. Finally Vern told the therapist he didn't want him to come back any more.

The physical therapist did insist that Vern needed a hospital bed, and he talked to Vern's primary care physician about it. The doctor Okayed it. I then contacted the doctor assigned to Vern at the VA hospital, and she said she would order it. When it never came I tried contacting her again by e-mail as she had requested. No answer. I tried again. No response. Frustrated I sent a letter to her mailing address asking if she'd ordered the bed. A few days later the letter was returned to me stamped, "No longer here. Take her off your list." The doctor had left the VA hospital, and no one took the time to notify us that we needed to be assigned to another doctor. Great!!

The one person from the home nursing company who really helped Vern was the Occupational Therapist, Cathy Barton. She was the person who suggested we try the bathrobe to dry him. She brought him a tray made with inch-high sides to help keep his dishes from sliding off as he tried to feed himself in the early stages. She was always thinking ahead to what might help him be as independent as possible. Vern looked forward to her coming, and really enjoyed her visits. She was good for him. They found so many things to talk about and that helped Vern a lot: and she cared about finding things in catalogs that might help make him more comfortable.

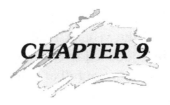

CHAPTER 9

As of August 1, 2009

List of things that Vern can no longer do .

Dry himself after his shower. I put the terry cloth bathrobe on him and dried his legs and feet while the bathrobe absorbed the water from his body.

Hold a newspaper or magazine

Shop

Shower alone

The occupational therapist brought him a bench for the tub so he could sit while I washed him.

The occupational therapist also brought him utensils with large handles to help him eat, and a thing to clip on the side of the plate to push his food up to so it wouldn't slide off the plate, and the food could go in the spoon or on the fork. These things felt clumsy to him, so I started feeding him myself.

He had to have a straw to drink liquids.

Vern's brother, Vic, his wife, Ann, and their son, Eric, flew in from Cincinnati on August 22nd. As we all sat around visiting, Vern began telling Vic, who was younger by ten years, stories about their parent's struggles as a young married couple. Ann decided to record some of these stories, and later, she made CD's that she shared with the rest of the family, - a great way to preserve the voice and stories of a loved one. This extreme generosity on Ann's part was appreciated by all of us.

By the middle of August the word had gotten out about how disabled Vern was and the visitors really started pouring in, all people whose lives he'd touched over the years. Every day, and I mean every day, we had a house full of company. Vern was a very popular guy. One day when Mary came to clean the house with her helper, Vern apologized for the house being so messy from all the company.

She answered, "Your house is always the cleanest house we clean."

I was in the process of finishing up painting the outside of the house. It was a project that Pat and I had started a few months earlier on one side, and Derek and I were doing the rest of it. Derek did the ladder parts, allowing me to do the lower parts, because he didn't want me to fall. I had just a little bit of yellow paint left to complete the job and went out to finish while Mary cleaned the house.

When I came back in after finishing the paint job, I said, Mary, I really appreciate what you do around here, because I just wouldn't be able to keep up. My whole routine has changed since Vern got sick."

"That's because you are a caregiver now."

I had never thought of it that way. Even though I had taken care of my mother after her heart attack for several months, and at other times, as she had several health problems before I eventually had to put her in a nursing home. I had also taken care of Vern's father for almost seven years. At those times I did truly feel like a caregiver. But for some reason taking care of Vern, who was worse off than either of them, I just never thought of it as being a caregiver until Mary said it out loud and then I realized she was right.

On August 15, 2009, we were officially notified by mail that the VA found Vern to be 100 % disabled. To look at him you couldn't tell. We had company the middle of August, and our friend said, "He's doing well isn't he?"

I answered, "No." That's all I could say, because it was too hard for me to explain.

By that time he was unable to put wood in the stove, he needed help to walk anywhere, even to the bathroom.

September 2, we took another trip to the UWMC for more tests. We knew Vern's lungs were getting weaker. The doctor said, "Probably in six months you will need a breathing apparatus at night to help you breathe. I want to see you in six months to discuss the breathing problems and you need to see our pulmonary doctor at the same time."

She also emphasized that he needed a wheelchair, and a recliner with a headrest. She gave me a list of things I needed to get to help in my care-giving duties.

Mechanisms for personal hygiene with toileting

A waist belt for assistance with his walking to prevent falls

A lift chair -- it is a device to help lift the patient when they cannot get out of the chair by themselves.

Grab bars for the shower

And the power wheelchair.

I contacted Mike Webb, our Veteran's advocate, to talk to him about finding a VA doctor at the Federal Way VA Clinic rather than having to drive to Ft. Lewis Army Base hospital.

He told us, "Federal Way VA Clinic is where I go for my medical needs and I am happy with them. It is a nice new clinic and the people are friendly."

I called and made an appointment for Vern to see a Nurse

Practitioner. The doctors all had full schedules.

Early in September the occupational therapist was ready to discharge Vern from her services. In order for us to have someone to turn to, she contacted Sonja Zimmer of the Evergreen Chapter of ALS. They set up a meeting at our home when they could both be present and we could meet Sonja.

The ALS doctor had given me a list of things Vern needed. On September 10th, the occupational therapist and Sonja arrived for our meeting. We had a discussion about that list of things. We exchanged a lot of information with each other. Sonja told us where we could buy a transport chair, lift chair, and a bidet for the toilet in the laundry room that Vern always used. Those were the things on the list from the doctor.

The bidet was one of the best suggestions made to us, as Vern was having so much trouble with his hands that he was having difficulty wiping himself, even with baby wipes. The bidet is an add-on to the toilet seat and fits on a regular toilet. When activated, it cleans with a flow of water and dries with air.

The nearest place for us to go for a bidet was Sequim, WA. Sirena drove us. It took nearly all day for us to get there and back, but we did buy a portable bidet. It was well worth the effort and expense.

Giving Vern control again was huge. Once he had the bidet, there was only one problem. That was the day he couldn't manage the remote control, and he hit the enema button instead of the posterior button to wash.

He told that story to anyone who would listen, about how much that water shooting up there shocked him and hurt. He'd laugh as he told the story. He never lost his sense of humor right up until the last few weeks of his life.

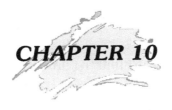

CHAPTER 10

Knowing we were soon going to need a wheelchair ramp, Vern and Derek measured and purchased cedar lumber for it. Vern wanted it to match the wood of the sunroom he built, so that it wouldn't look like an "add-on" to the house. He was a perfectionist in all he did, so he didn't want the ramp to look out of place. Today, many people walk right by it and don't even think of it as the wheelchair ramp until I point it out to them. It truly does look like part of the house.

Over a period of three days I stained the lumber, and Derek, under Vern's instructions from a chair, built the foundation for the ramp. Once the wood was dry, Vern instructed Derek about how to finish the ramp.

We had been told that Veteran's Affairs would reimburse us. When I gave a list of the materials to the social worker at the VA hospital they told us they wouldn't pay for it because we hadn't asked permission first.

By the middle of October I was noticing a weight loss in Vern: first in his shoulders, and arms, then his butt, and finally it was beginning to be noticeable in his face. I asked him one day when I was cleaning him up, "You told me you would divorce me if I weighed more than you. Does that still hold true?"

His response was, "You've got me over a barrel now."

It was hard finding a time to get my hair cut. I finally made an appointment and told my hairdresser, "Cut it short because it is driving me crazy and I just don't have time to come in as often as I should."

With surprise in her voice she asked, "Do you want a neck cut like mine?"

"Yes," I said, "I just can't find the time to get in here with taking care of Vern."

She again asked if I wanted it as short as hers. I answered, "Yes, let's go for it."

My hair is naturally curly so it curls up easily. When she finished she was so excited and said, "Oh, Delores, that's the best hair cut I ever did for you. I just love it!"

It felt good, and I knew it would be easy to take care of. When I walked in the door, Vern said, "Where's your hair? You don't have much left!"

I answered, "It will grow out."

He never liked my hair cut short, and until it grew out he kept making comments like, "Don't take too long to comb your hair," or "You forgot to put your wig on today."

That went on for weeks; finally I got tired of it and said, "Well, I have more hair than you do." I hated to say that to him because he'd always been so proud of his beautiful hair.

On November 9, 2009, I received a call from the Veteran's Hospital at Ft. Lewis setting up a time for us to get Vern measured for a motorized wheelchair. When they told me the appointment was at 9:00 A.M. on December 15th I stated, "Oh! That is much too early."

Having to get a man showered, shaved, and dressed, get myself ready, and travel for an hour in order to arrive by 9:00 seemed impossible at the time. And we didn't know if we would have snow on the ground. They informed me that was the only time of the day that they did those types of appointments, so we did it. Vern desperately needed the wheelchair by that time.

Each week seemed to present a new problem. By the middle of November, I could no longer get his jeans on him. He hated sweat pants, on anybody, so refused to buy them for himself. Instead, I purchased several pairs of nice pajamas from Nordstrom's Rack. He lived in them most of the time, unless he had a doctor's appointment. I would iron them so he looked nice, "My own Hugh Hefner".

We purchased a speaker phone because Vern couldn't hold a phone, and he had many people calling him. Before we got the speaker phone someone had to hold the phone to his ear and that bothered him, especially if it was a long conversation. The speaker phone was a blessing for all of us.

It was also in the middle of November that the Occupational Therapist discharged Vern from her services. She had helped us as much as she felt she could. She left it up to Sonja Zimmer to take over for our needs in the future. We had grown much attached to Cathy, and hated to think we might not see her again, but she said she'd keep in touch, and she was true to her word.

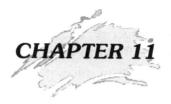

CHAPTER 11

Each year I do a Christmas letter. It is more like a newspaper, so it takes me a while to put it together. As I was working on it at the end of November, Vern told me, "I don't think I will be around next Christmas to see your letter."

"I hope you are calculating that wrong," I answered. "I've rather enjoyed taking care of you: it's like playing with a doll. I can dress you any way I want to, comb your hair any way I want, give you a bath, shave you, tuck you into bed and cover you up, just like a doll." We both laughed.

Our friend, Inge, joined us for Thanksgiving dinner, Vern really enjoyed it, but he did feel bad because I had to feed him, and he was afraid my food would be cold by the time I got around to eating it. I told him I've fed a lot of babies, so I was used to eating cold food. Besides, I could always warm it up in the microwave oven."

Derek and I were in the family room and I heard a glass fall on the kitchen floor. I ran in to see if Vern was all right. He had tried to get himself a drink of water rather than asking us to get it for him, and he dropped it. I couldn't help but laugh because if someone else had done that he would have been furious.

It was like taking care of a one or two year old who wanted to be independent but wasn't ready to be. I didn't want to tell him that, because I knew it would hurt his feelings, so instead I said, "You said the house was going to be dirty when Mary comes on Friday to clean. You just want to make sure the floor is clean." He made many messes that I had to clean up because he didn't want to ask for help.

The lift chair we ordered came the first part of December. We couldn't order it with a swivel because of the mechanism on the bottom that makes it lift. Vern, being stubborn and creative in his thinking, decided he could figure out a way to make a swivel for the chair. He was not about to sit and face one way in the living room. He'd always been able to turn around and watch the wild birds and squirrels we feed, and he wanted to still be able to do that. He figured out what was needed and instructed Derek how to do it. He was thrilled about that swivel.

Derek and I had put the artificial Christmas tree up in the sunroom. Our neighbor Debbie Pedersen and her daughter Angie came over and decorated it for me, allowing me to work more on my Christmas letter. When they finished, all of us had hot chocolate and cookies. Vern was able to turn in his chair to see the decorated tree in the sunroom.

Vern continued to get weaker in December. I would be feeding him, and suddenly his head would just drop down because his neck muscles were weak. It made it very difficult for him to eat. We eventually put a soft neck brace on him to hold his head up.

December 15th arrived, just one year to the day of his fall on the icy sidewalk. It found us heading to Ft. Lewis to have him measured for his motorized wheelchair.

The procedure took much longer than we ever expected. He was to get a wheelchair with a joy stick for him to steer it. The VA occupational therapist who measured him for the chair could see he was failing fast. She insisted that we apply for a hospital bed for him and that we apply for a grant to remodel the house because he might hit a plateau where he'd stay for a long time. She also told us to fill out paperwork for partial payment for a vehicle that would accommodate the wheelchair. Sirena suggested that we use public transportation that is made for that. We all agreed that was a better solution.

This occupational therapist told us she wouldn't be ordering the wheelchair for probably two months because she had jury duty and a vacation after that coming up. That worried me because of Vern's rapid decline.

We were having a hard time trying to convince ourselves that we needed to modify the home we had built to accommodate the motorized wheelchair. We finally decided that once we got the wheelchair, we would make any changes needed, hoping to do it without tearing the house up.

The next day Vern could not get off his bidet and I had to lift him. I thanked God that I was strong enough. I also had to lift him to a sitting position to get him out of bed in the mornings. Before that, he used to kick his legs, trying to force himself into a sitting position. But in doing so he jarred his brain, very much like a baby who has been shaken, and it caused him to have dizzy spells. When he mentioned this to his doctor, he was told to stop doing that, and was given medication for the dizziness. His legs became so weak he would not have been able to do it much longer, anyway.

About this time, Vern decided he wanted to try sleeping in his lift chair at night. I spent the night on the davenport beside him, but neither of us slept. Since that didn't work, he asked me to sleep with him in his bed, so I could turn him and cover him up when he got cold, and move his legs, and arms when it got so painful lying in one position.

For years, Vern had gotten up sometime during the night because of pain in his shoulder. Since he hadn't wanted to disturb me, he usually ended up sleeping on the sofa or in the other bedroom, so spending a whole night in bed together was a change for us.

His body jerked and twitched so much that neither of us slept well there, either. He was constantly waking me just as I dozed off, telling me to move his arms, his legs, and to turn him. That was an especially difficult time for both of us because neither of us was getting proper sleep.

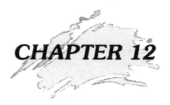

CHAPTER 12

Just before Christmas I bought Vern three new dress shirts at Costco. He was furious with me. "I'll never live long enough to wear them. I hope Derek likes them."

I told him, "I'm tired of dressing you in the same old shirts all the time, especially when I take you for appointments." Many times he got compliments on how nice his new shirts looked, so I think others must have gotten tired of his old shirts too.

People still came to visit every day, and one day we had 15 people. That evening he wanted me to give him another shower. He stated, "It is sometimes so tiring to have that much company all at once. It's just nice to have quiet time tonight."

December 29th I fed him pancakes, sausage, an egg, and juice for breakfast. When he was through eating he said, "If I had to die, now would be a good time, because I'm warm, content, and full from a great breakfast."

I told him, "Don't say that. It is too close to the first of the month, and your checks will be coming in." I chuckled.

"Yes, I thought about that too," he said. That's what keeps me going." Actually I think it was his ability to find humor in his condition that kept him going.

Sirena had borrowed our pickup, and when she returned it, I took her home. It was New Year's Eve, and she told me, "If you ever need someone to stay with Dad while you do yard work, shopping or anything, and I'm not working, I'll be happy to come have coffee with him while you do that."

I don't recall ever calling on her to do that because Vern wanted to know where I was and what I was doing every minute, but an offer like that is so helpful to caregivers. Derek and I did go shopping a few times when Mary was cleaning our home, but the rest of the time I was right there.

We met with the Nurse Practitioner for the first time at the Federal Way Veteran's Clinic on January 13th. Again, we took Sirena with us. Since she is an RN we thought that having her with us whenever possible at these types of appointments was important.

When the Nurse Practitioner called us back to her office she said the staff told her, "There's a team out here waiting to see you." From then on they referred to us as "The Team."

The Nurse Practitioner was so much better than the doctor we had at Ft. Lewis who disappeared. She spent two hours with us, putting information in the computer about Vern. Altogether it was as if we were starting all over again, but at least she got things moving, and she was only ten minutes away.

She discovered nothing had been done on the wheelchair order, which we knew was a strong possibility, and she ordered Vern's medication through the VA and had it mailed to us.

We discussed the need of a hospital bed. I was still sleeping with Vern turning, covering and moving his limbs all night long, which meant I didn't get much sleeping done. Just as I'd start to doze off he'd tell me to move his head, arms, or legs. It was wearing both of us out. I told her that it was supposed to have been ordered much earlier by Vern's primary physician but no one ever seemed to follow through. She said she'd be happy to work with Vern's primary physician, and would get the bed ordered.

Vern's hands had been swelling and curling up as the muscles contracted, and they were very painful. I had been putting ice packs on them to help relieve the pain, and keep the swelling down. The nurse practitioner ordered braces for him to lay his arms and hands in, which would help keep his fingers straight, and she told me to continue using the ice packs.

At one point she asked Vern what his condition was at present. He listed his many problems and added, "Other than that I'm 100%."

We all laughed, and I said, "You're 100% all right, Vern, but 100% the wrong way."

When I told Sonja Zimmer what Vern had said, and that he still had a sense of humor she responded, "Oh my! The ups, downs, trials and tribulations of living with ALS. Thank goodness for a sense of humor!"

Near the end of January, I was building a fire in the wood stove and had gone out to get the firewood from the sunroom to put in the stove. When I walked back in the main part of the house, Vern was frantically calling my name.

I rushed into the bedroom and said, "That was a pretty frantic call," and chuckled to lighten the moment since I didn't see anything seriously wrong. He replied grumpily "Well, that was the eighth time I called for you. I felt like I was in a nursing home where I've heard people call 'Nurse! Nurse!' and no one comes."

My immediate thought was about the poor nurses in a hospital or nursing home that have four or more patients assigned to them, trying to care for them, and keep them happy, maybe even a critical patient or two. Here I was unable to keep one patient happy - and he was my husband.

At the end of January, the hospital at Ft Lewis called us to make an appointment for Vern to try out different controls for the wheelchair. Sirena wasn't available to go with us, but Derek was. We didn't want to miss the appointment because it was frustrating to see Vern deteriorate so fast, and the wheelchair process seemed to be moving too slowly.

In the short period of time since we had first seen the nurse practitioner, Vern had lost all mobility in his hands, and could only move his head. The motorized wheelchair that was finally ordered had a head control to fit him. He got to pick the color, forest green.

It was the first case of ALS that this group had dealt with, and they didn't realize the urgency in getting things done for an ALS patient. They had no sense of the fast decline these patients have verses a long term patient.

We were told the wheelchair should be ready in two months, making it due in March. Vern was really looking forward to it, so he could get out in the fresh air and go see the neighbors as they were working in their yards. As my friend, Marjorie said, "The dream of freedom dies hard. To a guy, nothing says freedom like a motorcycle: or in Vern's case, a beautiful dark green motorized wheelchair"

He had always walked around the neighborhood each day, after feeding his animals. He missed that so much. At the same time, the many trips to his doctor's appointments were exhausting him. Mostly he just wanted to stay home and rest and catnap.

Ann sent me the book "Tuesdays With Morrie." by Mitch Albom The story is about a former student hearing on TV that a professor he had in college now had ALS. He looked him up and visited him every Tuesday until his death. As I read the book, and about Morrie's struggles, realized yes, that was what we were living with every day. Ann is very good about sending me books that are appropriate to whatever is happening in my life at the moment.

Many people suggested we take a trip: go somewhere that we'd always wanted to see. But neither one of us had the energy to even think about the hassle that would involve.

We'd done a lot of traveling earlier in our lives. We had visited Mexico, Canada and every state in the United States, and when he was in the Army stationed in Germany for two years, he saw a lot of Europe. Now, what he liked best was being at home, able to relax and doze off when he felt like it. As for me, I couldn't imagine traveling with ALS.

February the 4th was when we were scheduled to have Vern's breathing assessed. The doctor told him his breathing tests showed he needed a breathing apparatus. A tracheotomy was also suggested, but Vern refused when the doctor told him it wouldn't give him a better quality of life, only prolong his dying. The doctors told him that seventy-five percent of ALS patients choose not to have a tracheotomy.

I was feeding Vern, and he was having a lot of difficulty swallowing solid food because of the weakness in the muscles in his neck. The doctor suggested a stomach peg, which would allow for food to be placed directly into the stomach. At first Vern said no, but after he talked to my sister's husband, Jerry, who'd had one for six years, he relented.

The stomach peg would be useful, not just to provide nutrition, but because it would make it easier to give Vern his medications. It had to be inserted soon, while his breathing capacity would still allow it.

"What is the prognosis from here?" Vern asked the doctors.

"Without the breathing apparatus we think you will only have until next January."

Less than a year.

The next time Derek and I went to Costco, I was looking at the men's socks, because the washing machine seemed to have a sock eating monster, and I needed to replace the missing ones. I knew which ones were his favorites, so I put two packages of five in the cart.

Derek looked at me very seriously, and said, "Mom, don't buy too many green bananas."

As cruel as it sounds we both burst out laughing. I knew exactly what he meant. He didn't need to explain.

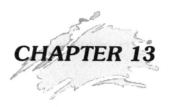

CHAPTER 13

I'd begun writing in my journal about the progress of Vern's disease almost every night when I went to bed. But, after I started having to take care of Vern's every need during the night, I seldom had the time to write.

When I put him in bed at night he began to complain about the weight of the bedding. It was only one sheet, and a light-weight blanket and this was early February. He complained that he felt like they were tangled up, and he would thrash around like a seal, trying to untangle bedding that wasn't tangled. I assumed it was the dying nerves that made him feel the covers were so cumbersome.

He also accused me of tucking the covers in on my side of the bed so that he couldn't turn over. I had to literally show him I had not tucked the covers in before he'd believe me.

It was, of course, his weak muscles that wouldn't let him turn over. He was miserable lying in one position for more than a few minutes, and I had to get out of bed in order to turn him over, -- many, many times during the night.

He couldn't move his head so I'd have to lift it and turn it as well as well as the rest of his body. He was in pain, and so was I, because I couldn't stop his pain. I also admit I got frustrated with his demands and my lack of sleep.

Derek was very diligent about keeping the bird feeders full, as well as peanuts in the squirrel feeding box. All were in Vern's view so he could watch the birds from his lift chair. Vern especially liked to see the pileated woodpeckers. They don't frequent the feeders as often as the other birds, so it is always a thrill to see them land on the trunk of the tree where the suet cakes are mounted.

On February ninth I wrote in my journal: "Turn the flowers so I can see the lilies." (Vern had been referring to a bouquet that our friend, Inge, had brought the day before.)

Continuing my notes in the journal, "Here it is in early February and Vern alerts me to the Hollywood Plum tree that is just starting to bud. I've been outside, not far from the tree, and did not even notice. He, in his lift chair, misses nothing that is going on in the back yard, whether it is the neighbor's kids playing or Mother Nature performing her magic.

Vern's cheeks and chin had kept soft by the everyday shaving. But, I was reminded of what an active outdoorsman he had always been as I touched his leathery forehead and massaged moisturizer into his dry skin - skin that was now flaking off. He commented 'My skin is dying before I do.' End of quote in my journal.

The progression of Vern's ALS seemed to be very fast from December to February. I didn't know if that was because it started in his arms and shoulders rather than his legs. No one had told us if he had a fast or slow type. We had been told that once it hits your arms and hands you have about three years, because it hits your lungs earlier than if it starts in your legs. Once it hits your lungs and you can no longer breathe, that is what kills you.

The neurologist at the VA hospital told us it is like freezing to death. The patient doesn't gasp for air. We exhale carbon dioxide as we breathe, but the patient with ALS doesn't exhale all the carbon dioxide. Once it has built up in your lungs, you just go to sleep and you don't wake up.

Vern had rejected the breathing apparatus that would help him breathe, which meant the carbon dioxide would build up faster. The doctor neither encouraged nor discouraged Vern about using the breathing apparatus. He just gave him the facts, telling him that only twenty-five percent of ALS patients choose to use it. Vern said later that it was very comforting to know how death would come.

On Valentine's Day, I dressed and shaved Vern, brushed his teeth and combed his hair, then helped him to the living room. I went in to the bathroom to put my makeup on, and I heard a loud, "DELORES!, DELORES!". I rushed into the living room to see what was wrong, and he said, "I will DISMISS you when I am through with you, REMEMBER THAT!!" He was serious, but I burst out laughing. It struck me so funny, that word "dismiss".

Then he added, "I don't know what I'm going to do when I lose my voice, I can't even ring a bell -- I couldn't even get a job at the Salvation Army." When I started to laugh again, he had to join in.

Sometimes though, despite the laughter, I was hurting inside. But I always knew he was hurting worse than I was. When friends would discuss with him how he felt about dying, he always answered, "I don't mind, because I've had a good life. But I want our friends and family to keep in touch with Delores once I'm gone, because she is going to need the emotional support." And then he'd get tears in his eyes.

The day after Valentine's Day, my friend, Marjorie, brought me some very special violets her grandmother had brought from England for me to plant in my flower beds, and I gave her some iris that I had dug up. She stayed and visited with Vern and me. We hadn't seen her for a while even though we've always kept in touch. Vern told me later how much he enjoyed that visit.

On February 16th after I had given Vern his shower, his right knee buckled as he was climbing out of the tub. He ended up straddling the edge of the tub. He insisted I put him back in the tub and then lift him out. I told him, "Vern, common sense tells me that won't work. I don't think I can lift you out of the tub." He was determined that I try. As I was attempting it, he fell on top of me. Once I managed to get out from under him, I couldn't pick him up. He was just dead weight, unable to help me. He weighed about 160 pounds at the time, roughly thirty pounds heavier than I was, as he'd already lost a lot of weight. As I tried to pick him up, he kept slipping out of my arms and hands because his body was wet. It was like trying to pick up a large wet fish. I tried drying him off, but I still couldn't pick him up.

I called our neighbor, Eric Pedersen, who came and helped me. He isn't very big either, so I put the webbed belt around Vern's chest, Eric got behind him and we both lifted him and got him into the bedroom and on the bed where I could finish drying him off. I was so thankful for Eric's help!

The next day was Derek's day off, so he helped me with bathing Vern, but we all knew the showers were coming to an end. Instead, I started giving him sponge baths. He said they weren't as bad as he had thought they would be, because he'd worried he wouldn't feel as clean as he did after having a shower.

Vern had never had much patience, and as time went by, and he was more and more dependent, he became more and more impatient with Derek and me, especially over simple things. I knew it was because he was frustrated with himself, so I'd try to find a way to joke about whatever the problem was that was upsetting him, and sometimes those problems seemed absurd to me.

One time I was brushing his teeth and he wanted a particular tooth brushed just when he wanted it brushed and not when I was going to get to it. Often, he got impatient with me if we had conflicting ideas of what he needed at any particular moment. I'm sure that having me do all his personal hygiene was embarrassing to him, and that was what made him short-tempered.

About that time, he was also having trouble aiming when he went to the bathroom, because he couldn't hold his hands steady. I purchased extra pajama bottoms for him. Then I realized I needed to help him. At first I felt a little strange doing the aiming for him, but I knew it was something I needed to do. It was just another result of the disease that I needed to take care of, because he couldn't. It went with the job.

Late in February our water bill shot up twice as high as it should have been, and we discovered it was due to a leak in the pasture. Vern worried about it all night, knowing he could do nothing about it. He'd always been the guy in charge, but that was no longer true. Derek checked it out and managed to fix it the next day. When Vern knew it was fixed, he started to cry.

I went to him and gave him a hug, and he said gruffly, "I don't need your coddling." I found it strange that he used the term "coddling." I'd never heard him ever use that term in the fifty-seven years we'd been married. Perhaps it was the ALS talking.

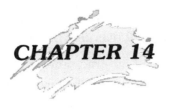

CHAPTER 14

By February 19, 2010, I was having health issues of my own. At this point, or even earlier, I should have asked for more help, but I thought I was doing okay with Derek and Sirena helping me. Derek came over every morning, staying with us until he had to go to work at 2:00. Sirena was wonderful about driving us to doctor and hospital appointments and helping me handle her father. But, the majority of Vern's care fell on me, and eventually, my body paid the price for all the lifting I'd been doing.

My problems included difficulty walking and a hernia. I had permanent damage that was going to require surgical repair. I worried about mentioning it to Vern because I didn't know who would take care of him during my surgery or my recovery period. I knew it was going to be major surgery, and that was a huge problem. I made an appointment with my doctor, and she referred me to a surgeon. She told the surgeon she wanted him to check me over and see if he could do something besides surgery because I told her I couldn't take time for surgery. I was hoping he could do a temporary repair until Vern passed away and then do the surgery.

My doctor gave me suggestions to help relieve my problems like breathing OUT when lifting, as weight lifters do, using my leg muscles rather than put strain on my abdominal muscles. The appointment with the surgeon was in two weeks.

The following evening as I was lifting Vern off the bidet his legs gave out and he fell to the floor. Thankfully Derek was still here and helped me pick him up. When the patient can't help you, it is like trying to lift a baby who hasn't learned to use his muscles to help but this baby weighed over one hundred sixty pounds.

February 28th rolled around and it was our fifty-seventh wedding anniversary. Yes, we got married as teenagers. He was nineteen and I was eighteen. I wrote in my journal, "And from what the doctors say, it may be our last."

Mary and her husband, Jay, surprised us by bringing us an anniversary cake with a studio picture of us when we had been married five years. Desiree, three months old, was in the original picture, but somehow the bakery had cropped her out of the picture, so it was just the two of us on the cake.

Mary had taken the picture to work and asked the girls if they recognized the people on the cake. Most of them had been here one time or another to help Mary clean our home. No one knew, but they all said they thought it was a picture of movie stars. Oh how we change as we get older.

I asked Mary and Jay if I could freeze the cake until Desiree, Gene, Cole and Tess came from New York, because we were going to celebrate our anniversary with them the following month. They agreed.

The first of each month, Vern would get his veteran's disability check and his social security check. Upon waking the morning of March 1, he said, "Well, I lived long enough to get another pay check."

Later in the day I was feeding him kettle corn as a snack and he asked me, "Is that all you have to do is feed this little bird?"

I told him, "Yes."

When I finished he said, "That was pretty good. I should get paid more often than just once a month."

He wasn't always so cheerful. One evening I was taking my

medication and he said, "I'm going to the bathroom."

I said, "Okay." finished swallowing my pills, and walked into the bathroom behind him.

He yelled at me, "When I say I'm going to the bathroom I want you to know and remember it isn't a one man operation!"

While Sirena was here one day he told her, "I need to blow my nose." She grabbed a tissue and took it to him, and as she walked away he reminded her he needed more than a tissue. He needed her to help him blow his nose.

Later I was getting a drink of water and he called for me, I went in the bedroom to see what he needed. He told me, "I want you to brush my teeth." and then he added, "When I want something, I want you hooked to my hip." It sounds funny but he was serious. Sometimes I just wanted to laugh because at times he was so unreasonable. I often wondered if his behavior was a result of the ALS or if it was just truly his personality.

One time he even got mad at Sirena. The three of us were going to the grocery store. As we were getting ready to leave the house, I lost a battery out of my hearing aid. Sirena stopped to help me look for it. Vern ended up standing on the wheelchair ramp longer than he found acceptable. He got very upset and yelled at her. That surprised me because Sirena was his favorite child and everyone knew it. He never hid the fact. When we got to the commissary he didn't want to come in with us, and Sirena and I talked about how upset he'd gotten with her. Then she asked, "Mom, if he got that upset with ME what is he like with you and Derek?"

I answered, "He has NO patience with us."

We reached the car after shopping and were surprised to see him sitting sideways with the car door open. It turned out that although we'd rolled the windows down, he still got hot. He managed to get the attention of a young woman who opened the door for him and helped him move his legs. Needless to say, he was angry when we got to the car, and he complained about it for days, to anyone who would listen. Sirena called Desiree in New York about the incident, telling her "I almost killed Dad."

Sirena reminded me of the time a month earlier when we had gone to the commissary to shop. Vern had still been able to go into the store in the transport chair. As we came out to the parking lot afterward, Sirena hit the remote button to open the trunk of the car. It wouldn't open and he told her, "Push the button."

She said, "I did, Dad."

He told her, "Well, push it again."

This went on a few times with him getting louder and louder, until he yelled, "Push the damn button!"

I was getting embarrassed, and turned around to see if anyone was watching us, and I saw our car in the row behind us with the trunk lid open. Someone with a car identical to ours was parked in a handicapped spot one row away from our car. We all had to laugh.

Despite his impatience with Derek and me, Vern's social interactions with other people were wonderful. He always seemed upbeat to them. Everyone loved him and thought he was such a saint, but when it was just Derek and me, the communication was completely different. Still, I couldn't help but feel sorry for him even as grumpy as he got, because he had lost so much. I could well understand his frustrations as the disease was rapidly depriving him of his dignity and life.

Morgan, Erika and Nathaniel had been over one day to mow the lawns, and the pasture and clean the barn. Vern asked me to get his wallet and pay them. As I was getting the money out, I accidentally pulled out a studio picture of me that was taken in the mid 1970's. I had no idea he carried it in his wallet and for that many years.

I said, "Oh! Who is this?"

His response was, "She's been running shotgun with me for a long time."

This reminded me of the many times we'd gone hunting around the hills in the Grand Coulee area. He'd drive over those old, bumpy, dangerous roads and we'd almost roll the car. Yes, that was really riding shotgun.

I commented, "And she intends to keep on doing it."

That hadn't always been easy, even before he was diagnosed with Lou Gehrig's Disease. Vern's mother had warned me when we were dating that he was never happy unless he had a pretty woman on each arm and that never changed throughout our marriage. But we had gotten through those many ups and downs, and now, I put all that aside in order to help him get through this horrible disease.

He was in pain, and hated not being in charge any more. He was unable to even care for himself, and having to be completely dependent on others was killing him in more ways than one. Each day I wondered how I could lighten his burden so he'd look forward to the next day.

I had another appointment with my surgeon in early March. The method he'd tried to temporarily alleviate my problems didn't work. He said surgery was necessary and the sooner the better. I knew he was right.

The family and I discussed my surgery and we decided what our schedules would be if I were to have it done as soon as possible. We decided we would have to hire someone to come in and take care of Vern for a while. Sirena said she'd take two weeks off of work, stay with her dad all day, and help me when I needed it. Derek would take time off work as well. And we would hire someone to come in three hours in the evenings. We figured that would work, as I had always recovered fast after surgery.

Vern was also going to have the surgery to place the stomach peg. We were hoping the wheelchair would come soon, since he was going to need to stay in the hospital for five days learning how to use it. The hospital staff suggested we schedule that and the surgery at the same time. That way, the nurses could watch the surgical site and see that it didn't get infected. If I could schedule my surgery while he was in the hospital, it would be less stress on everyone.

Unfortunately, the wheelchair didn't arrive in time, and I had a hard time contacting the surgeon to set up my surgery. Vern was scheduled to have his stomach peg surgery March 24th so we had to work around that. Desiree's family was to come on March 27th, and I didn't want my surgery before that.

On March 16th, my brother-in-law called to tell me my sister, Alzada, passed away in her sleep during the night. She had been suffering with bone cancer, and I worried about her, but there was nothing I could do as she lived in Maine and we lived in Washington State. The cancer had been discovered in early September, and she'd had chemo for a while, but opted to stop when it made her so sick. She'd been under Hospice care since the first part of March. My sister's death left me the last one living in my birth family. My father and two of my brothers also died of cancer. Alzada was 76. Life really is so fragile.

A couple days after my sister passed away, one of our visitors and I were talking about dreams of our departed ones, and she asked Vern "to come back and keep in touch with us." He said he would.

I've had other people tell me they'd come back and keep in touch with me after they passed away. None of them ever did, though I've had very vivid dreams of family that have passed away. When I woke up, it was as if they really had visited me. Did it really happen or was it just a dream? I don't know. It seemed so real at the time.

I have a hearing problem, and later in the evening, Vern was talking to me and I misunderstood what he said. I asked him, "When you come back to visit and talk to me, will you please talk plainly enough so I can understand you?"

He answered, "I'll get up real close to your ear." We both chuckled.

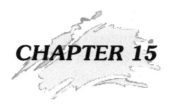

CHAPTER 15

During our marriage, Vern would never tell me he loved me. One night as I was putting him to bed he said, "Thank you for taking care of me; I love you." I was so surprised that he actually said these words to me. I was always sure in his own way that he did, because early in our marriage I had filed for divorce. At first he refused to sign the papers. Then when things between us were getting no better I asked him again to sign the papers and he agreed. We got to the attorney's office and I signed the papers, he picked up the pen, looked at the papers, looked at me, looked back at the papers, looked at me again, threw the pen down and said, "I'm not signing them." And walked out of the office, leaving the attorney and me both standing there with our mouths open.

So even though he found he couldn't say the words, I think he must have loved me. I gave him opportunities to leave, but he always came back.

March 31st, Derek decided to take the garbage to the dump, and I was gathering everything up for him. Vern said, "There's that very sexy lady, getting the garbage."

I turned and asked him, " Why did you say that?" Many years ago he called me his sexy babe, but he hadn't called me sexy for many years. I didn't understand what brought that up.

He responded by telling me that when one of the neighbors, Kellie Lee, had been here the day before and I walked out of the room, she leaned over to him and whispered in his ear, "She's really a very sexy lady." So I knew he was teasing me.

Vern's pain had become unbearable, especially at night, so the doctor prescribed a stronger pain medication. By the time March 24th rolled around and Vern was due to have his stomach peg put in, he couldn't sit very long. At the hospital, we had waited over an hour, and Vern couldn't stand sitting in his transport chair even though we had cushions in it. He told me to go to the front desk and tell them he needed a bed.

I did as he said. The lady at the desk got on the phone and very sternly said, "I have Mrs. Warner at the front desk and she said her husband has Lou Gehrig's Disease and can't sit any longer. He needs a bed NOW!

In less than three minutes, a nurse came and got him and took him back. I went with them, got him undressed, and into in a gown, and put him to bed. Then the nurse told me I had to leave because another patient was coming in. Vern told the nurse to send Sirena and me home because we'd been there so long already, and it was going to be another two hours before his surgery.

We left, stopping at the store to buy me a new pair of jeans. Sirena insisted that I needed new jeans because the others were so faded and didn't have much life left in them. I hadn't been shopping for ages, except to go to the grocery store. I bought a couple pairs of jeans, and the first time I put a pair on, a neighbor who was stopping by the house said, "You got new jeans!"

I replied, "Gee, were my others really that bad? Is it so obvious I got new jeans?" and we both chuckled.

Sirena and I also stopped at a restaurant to pick up soup and sandwiches. We took them to Derek's house. He was preparing his guest room for Desiree's family's visit. We ate lunch, then we all worked together to help him finish up what needed to be done. He's a great housekeeper, so it didn't take much.

After I got home, I called the hospital to see how Vern was

doing. They said he had just gotten out of the operating room, and hadn't gotten to his room yet. They gave me his room number and his phone number. I wrote all the information down. About an hour later as I was fixing flowers in a vase, it hit me he couldn't answer the phone. He couldn't even talk on the phone unless it was a speaker phone. What was I thinking?

Sirena called and suggested that I contact the hospital and tell them Vern wouldn't be able to use the call button because of his ALS. When I called they said they had pinned the call button to his pillow, so that he could roll his head onto it if he needed them. The nurses even took time to feed him what he could manage to eat.

I called the hospital to see how Vern did during the night, and I was lucky to get the nurse who had taken care of him. She said he'd had a very restless night and she had to readjust him several times during the night. I thought that wasn't any different than at home. I was hoping the hospital bed would make him more comfortable.

Both the nurses and Vern told us that sometimes he'd have them come and turn him, and before they'd even get out the door he'd have them come back and readjust him. He felt bad about that but said he was just so uncomfortable.

Derek and I picked him up in the afternoon. We were shown a video of how to take care of the surgical site and how to use the stomach peg and were asked if we had any questions before they discharged him.

When we picked him up we found out he'd had no pain medication after surgery. Unbelievable! The surgeon had not ordered any, and when the nurse tried to call the doctor no one could reach him. No wonder he was uncomfortable! The day nurse went to the head doctor and complained about that. It took a long time to get checked out, and when we got him home, we gave him pain medication, and again when he went to bed. He only woke me up three times during the night. The best night's sleep we'd had in months.

By the next day, he was showing his stomach peg off to anyone who wanted to see it, just like he had his bidet when we got it.

While I was giving him a sponge bath the next morning he said, "You've been so good all this time."

I expected him to go on to explain why he said that, but he didn't so I answered, "Of course. You are my husband and I love you."

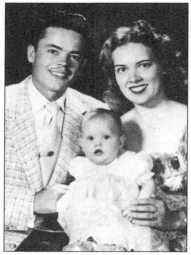

Vern, Delores and baby, Desiree. This is the photo that they put on the 57th anniversary cake.

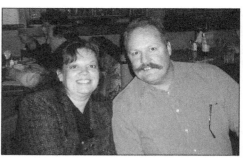

Sirena and Patrick.

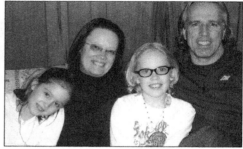

Tess, Desiree, Cole and Gene.

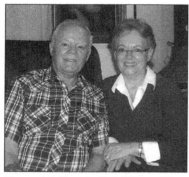

Vern and Delores on their 57th wedding anniversary. Vern died four months later
Photo by Mary North

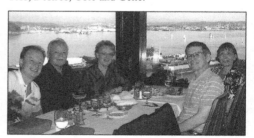

At the Warners' favorite restaurant, the Cliff House, in Tacoma, WA. Son, Derek, Vern, Delores, brother, Victor, and his wife, Ann.

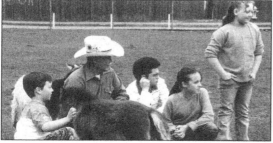

In healthier times: Grandson, Nathaniel, petting a new filly at the mini-farm, Papa Vern, grandson, Dustin, and granddaughters, Morgan and Erika.

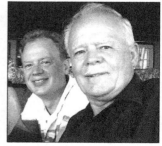

Derek and Vern.

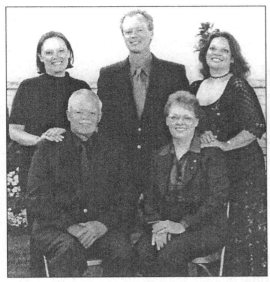

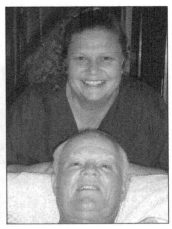

Vern with Tena Brown, bath aide.

This photo was taken as we celebrated our 50th wedding anniversary. Desiree, Derek, Sirena, Vern and Delores.

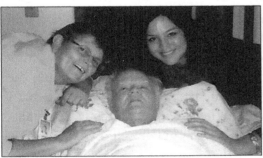

Hospice social worker Janine Carpenter, Vern and nurse Kelly Chumbley.

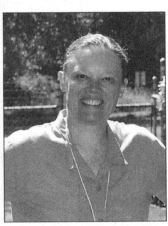

Desiree in 2010 while visiting Vern and Delores in Auburn, WA.

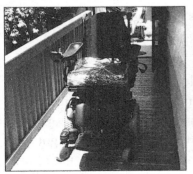

A specially made wheelchair that Vern was never able to use, sitting on the wheelchair ramp that Derek built.

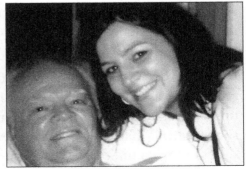

Vern and nurse Kelly Chumbley.

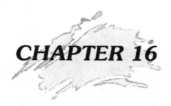

CHAPTER 16

Desiree's family arrived as expected. It was evening, and as I was feeding Vern, he got overly warm and wanted to go out to the sunroom. Soon, Derek, Desiree, and our ten year-old grandson, Cole, joined him. I was eating at the breakfast bar and I heard all this laughter coming from the sunroom. When I asked Desiree what they were laughing at, she said Cole had wanted to take a picture of his Papa with the cell phone, but the battery was dead. Vern told him, "It's okay, you'll be here for a while." Cole said, "Yes, but I'm afraid YOU won't be." Out of the mouths of babes.

April 1st, I had several tests done at the surgeon's office, and he scheduled my surgery for April 26th. He gave me the choice of types of surgery, and I opted for the type that didn't call for cutting the tendons in my abdominal area. The doctor said I made the right choice because I would heal faster. When I told Vern that I had chosen the other procedure he stated, "You made a mistake, you should have the abdominal surgery and have him cut out three inches of fat."

I never had three inches of fat to cut off, but he was always concerned about my weight. For years, he weighed me every other day to make sure I didn't weigh more than 120. He wanted me to stay at 118.

As I was weighing a patient at the doctor's office one day, a well-groomed, classy little lady, she told me she'd been married three times and not one of her husbands knew how old she was or what she weighed. That gave me courage the next time Vern got the scales out from under the bathroom sink, to reach down and put them back under the sink. I looked him in the eye and said, "You are more obsessed with my weight than I am. I'm not doing this anymore." He never got the scales out to weigh me again.

Sirena had gone with me to the surgeon's office and joined me as the doctor explained what needed to be done. He had to realign organs that had been rearranged by taking care of Vern. The repairs were going to be extensive. Afterward I briefly explained to the family what needed to be done, and our son-in-law, Gene said, "Sounds like a tune-up."

Sirena responded, "No, more like a major engine repair."

The hospital bed came when Desiree was still here visiting. We had it placed in the family room, then she and I went out and bought the bedding for it. That was a fun experience for us to do together. It had been a long time since we had an opportunity to go shopping. We found some good sales, so that made it even better.

One day during her visit, while Desiree was helping her dad get into his lift chair he complained that there was a lot of sensitivity around his stomach peg. She took a picture with her cell phone and sent it to Sirena and asked her why there was so much redness around it.

Sirena said she thought it was a pressure sore developing as it looked like the first stages of skin breakdown and told us to put 3x3 gauze bandages around the peg at the surgical site. That worked great.

While they were here, Gene took over the job of massaging Vern's hands and arms. Vern's hands were so painful when they were swollen and Gene relieved a lot of that by massaging them. Gene's hands were much stronger than mine and he could massage Vern's hands longer than I was able to.

When they flew back to New York on April 7th, there were a lot of tears at their departure. It was quite obvious it was going to be the last time they would see Vern alive and it was a hard goodbye.

So many tears.

By this time, Vern had reached the point where he could only drink liquids. We tried a nutrition supplement, but it gave him diarrhea. He could still walk well enough, with help, to make it to the toilet, and I got him there. But, I couldn't get him off the bidet. Derek had gone to work and I had to have our neighbor, Khieng Lee, come and help me lift him. Vern was embarrassed but Khieng is such a compassionate man: I was so thankful for his help.

I realized that I not only needed Derek and Sirena's help, now I was in need of added help, but, I would not put Vern in a nursing home. Vic and Ann called and offered to come and help, but I declined their offer. They had their own lives in Cincinnati.

Vern now had the hospital bed in our family room. Derek decided he would come after his swing shift and sleep on the sofa in the room with his dad and take care of him during the night so I could get some much needed sleep. It was April 11th I was back in my own bed for the first time in months, and it felt so good. I managed a full eight hours of sleep, although I woke several times expecting Vern to call me. Then I noticed he wasn't in bed with me and realized where I was and that Derek was with him, and rolled back over and went back to sleep. But, Derek didn't get much sleep.

After that, until Derek got off work at 11:00 pm, I would stay with Vern in the family room. Then I'd go to my bed, and Derek would take over his dad's care for the rest of the night. And believe me; he required a lot of care 24/7. The care giving never stopped.

Vern just couldn't get comfortable. At first, he could still kick his feet so he'd do that, and then want us to move his arms, his hands, his head, turn him over, and massage his body. Although his nervous system was withering away, he was in nearly constant pain.   It is tough to watch a person having to go through that. Even after he was paralyzed he still had a lot of pain. It's a horrible disease. Not all ALS patients have pain, but Vern had more than his share.

In April, we took Vern to the pulmonary physician at the VA hospital in Seattle. While I was waiting in line to check him in, I saw Sirena leave her dad in the transport chair and run to the room where they do vital signs. Then she came over to me, and I asked, "Is there a problem?"

She answered, "He can't breathe. I asked the nurse at vital signs to call someone and bring oxygen, and she said I had to talk to the woman at the check in counter, because she is new and didn't know what to do."

The gentleman ahead of me in line said, "If he can't breathe, that's not good." He pointed to our left, "Go over there and get someone."

Sirena rushed straight back to the physicians' area and grabbed a doctor, who told her the pulmonary physician would be coming any minute. The pulmonary physician did leave his patient and came to Vern immediately. I got out of line when I recognized the doctor who was headed toward Vern. The doctor was talking to him and Sirena frantically said to the doctor, "He needs oxygen!"

He responded, "We don't have any oxygen."

She questioned him, "Not even in the ER? No oxygen?"

"If we moved him to the ER we could give him oxygen. We couldn't believe what we were hearing. No oxygen in a pulmonary clinic? They wanted to put him in the hospital but he refused, so they rushed him to an area that was less crowded and much cooler. His breathing eased just from that. Sirena and I sat beside him worried he wouldn't make it, but he snapped out of it fairly quickly.

Vern then proceeded to go in to great detail with the doctor and his nurse about my up-coming surgery. I mean every detail, and when he finished I said, "That's probably more information than they cared to know." We all laughed and then Sirena added, looking at her dad, "There's a reason he's a pulmonary physician."

The doctor chimed in with, "I like working from the waist up." and we all laughed again.

We came home that day with a BiPap device, which is the mask used for sleep apnea. After attempting to use the BiPap, he found it very uncomfortable and asked if he could use the nose cannula. That worked much better for him.

The doctor also gave us a prescription to minimize Vern's pain and to keep the swelling in his hands down. It was supposed to have been given to him a long time before, but somehow the order slipped by the wayside. They forgot, however, to give him an order for oxygen.

At times in April and May I thought Vern was just giving up. That worried me, although I knew the real problem was that he was in so much pain. The Veteran's neurologist should have ordered pain medication much sooner, as he said he would, but, he'd somehow forgotten to. It was a major undertaking, trying to get the VA doctors to follow through with what they said they would do. We finally got the pulmonary physician to order new medication for him. Once he got that, he slept better and was much more comfortable, and that allowed both Derek and me to sleep better.

The day after the visit to Vern's pulmonary physician, Derek took his father to his primary care physician, who ordered oxygen sent to our home, and it was delivered the next day. The doctor told him, "Now is the time of your life when you can have whatever you want. If you want morphine, you can have it. Whatever you want you can have. His philosophy about end of life care was so much better than the Veterans Affairs doctors, and it was a great comfort to all of us.

While at the doctor's appointment, the doctor asked them if I had hired help in taking care of him. Vern answered, "No, my wife takes care of me."

The doctor asked, "Is she a BIG woman?"

Derek answered jokingly, "Yes, she weighs 250 pounds."

Vern didn't think it was funny.

The doctor suggested we sign up for Hospice, and said we should have signed up much earlier.

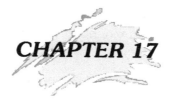

CHAPTER 17

We contacted a home health care facility about hiring help for Vern in the evenings while I would be recovering from my surgery. We were very specific about Vern's needs: to be fed, bathed, shaved and so on. We also said that we needed them to do minor house cleaning and laundry. The person we spoke with assured us that all of their staff were trained to do whatever we needed. We hired them to start the day of my surgery.

Derek and Sirena were both taking time off to help their dad while I was in the hospital, and to help take care of me if I needed help after I got home. The health care aide would come in for three hours in the evening to care for Vern.

My surgery took five and a half hours, much longer than the doctor had expected it to take, and I didn't recover as fast as I thought I would. I'm sure some of it was because I was rundown before I ever had the surgery. I usually recuperate fast, but not this time. Being age 75 didn't help matters either, though I've always been pretty active and healthy.

The nurses told me I had incisions in my groin area. They were still having problems getting my blood pressure up. The night nurse said she was going to call the doctor and talk to him. I asked her not to bother him in the middle of the night. She said, "That's what you're paying him the big bucks for." She called him, then came back to my room and said, "Yes, he wasn't very happy to be awakened in the middle of the night. Tough!"

As a result of her call, the doctor changed my pain medication to see if that would stop the nausea. It didn't, and I was in so much pain, and I couldn't keep food down.

When the doctor came in the next day to discharge me from the hospital, I was stunned. I was still vomiting, and I couldn't sit up in bed without pain because of the stitches and my blood pressure was still not normal. Still he sent me home. As I was preparing to leave, the certified nursing assistant caring for me suddenly remembered she could give me a "donut" to sit on and that helped tremendously. I wish I'd had it all along. I ended up sitting on it for weeks. The nausea continued for days, and a week after my surgery, I was still vomiting. I never dreamed I would be that sick.

The surgeon had ordered a physical therapist to work with me. When the physical therapist's office called me, I jokingly asked for a woman because they could see what a man had done to me. They sent a wife and husband who were both physical therapists to interview me and set up appointments. I ended up with the husband, because his wife was due to have a baby any day.

After the physical therapist showed me some exercises, I overdid them on my own, because I wanted to get well faster. My notes in my journal at that time are messy, very unlike my usual writing.

As I was getting stronger I went into the living room where Vern's health care aide was sitting on the sofa talking to him. I was surprised to see how sloppily she was dressed. She didn't even have her shoes tied, and here she was taking care of my very particular husband.

The next day, when my physical therapist came, he asked me to go into the kitchen and stand by the sink. I was appalled, when I stepped on the kitchen floor, to find it was sticky. There were three dirty dish cloths wadded up and thrown behind the faucet. They'd obviously not been rinsed out after being used. I told Vern that the aide, who by this time we were calling Ding-a-Ling, had to go.

Later, he told me that she hadn't been prepared to give him

sponge baths, or shave him, and when she fed him she spilled food all over his chest and clothing. She told us she had never done this type of work before. She had two sons: you'd think she'd know how to feed and bathe someone.

Sirena came over, and Vern and I were telling her how unhappy we were with the aide the agency sent us. Vern said they had also sent one other woman and a young man at different times. The woman told Vern she'd had MRSA and the young man was sent out with them telling him he was just to babysit Vern while I went out to get away from the care giving for a couple hours. Outrageous. I was still barely managing to get out of bed for a couple hours at that time.

When Sirena heard this she called the agency on the speaker phone. She and her dad told them not to send anyone out again; that we were going to find another home health care service. Sirena also told them she couldn't believe they'd send someone out who had had MRSA when her mother had just had major surgery and her dad was suffering from ALS. We'd heard that once you have MRSA bacteria you have a 98% chance of being a carrier. Vern and I were both immuno compromised. The agency knew that but still sent this person out to care for Vern.

The first week in May we signed up for Hospice care for Vern. I felt an urgency to get better because Vern had so little patience with others who were providing care for him, and it was embarrassing to me. I was starting to have less and less pain at this point, and only needing Tylenol a couple times a day.

We knew signing up with Hospice was the right decision when our Hospice nurse, Kelly Chumbley, came for her first visit.

She sat close to Vern in his lift chair interviewing him, and at one point she said, "Vern, am I too close to you?"

I answered for him, "A pretty girl too close to Vern? Are you kidding? It'll never happen." She laughed and so did Vern.

Nurse Kelly offered to sign Vern up for sponge baths with a Hospice aide, and he told her, "No, I don't have 'Ding-a-ling' trained yet."

When Vern told Kelly that, Derek and I really laughed because as upset with Ding-a-ling as he was, he still wanted to be in charge.

After we'd fired the first health care agency, we called another home health care service for evening care until I was able to take over again. They sent us a wonderful caregiver, who was trained. Tata Kamara had been here from Africa only eight years, and she was sweet, compassionate, and willing to work. She attended to Vern's needs while I rested in a lounge chair in the other room. She folded laundry, and she unloaded the dishwasher. Vern was never short tempered with the Hospice staff or Tata, and they provided wonderful care for him.

Since Vern could no longer cut his own toe nails and finger nails and they were so hard to cut, we had been taking him to Lynn's Nail Design salon who did that for him. When he was having so much trouble getting in and out of the car we asked if they would make a house call for him. and they did.

During my recovery, our neighbor, Debbie, who loves animals, took over the evening chores of feeding the horses, goats, peacocks, and chickens. She was a tremendous help while I was recuperating. She did it for a couple of months, every night as regular as could be. Sometimes her daughter, Angie, would help her. They would gather the eggs, and when Tata answered the door she would say to me, "It's the egg lady." Debbie, Angie and I have laughed about that ever since. When I first started moving around at home Debbie and Angie also helped get me to bed when Sirena wasn't here to help me. They were a blessing to us.

Sirena had thought she would be able to also take care of the animals, but once she got here and saw what all needed to be done, she was glad that she wasn't responsible for doing the chores outside as well as inside. She told me, "Many hands make light work."

While I was in the hospital, Vern declined to the point that he had to use the portable urinal. One of the first things I did when I was able to get up and around after surgery was to help him with that.

Nurse Kelly took over ordering Vern's medicine, because the VA wasn't very fast about getting it to him. She also ordered a bath aide, shave and shampoo for him starting the middle of May. That was such a relief to me, because I still wasn't able to do that after my surgery. Once the bath aide came we could see what a difference there was between a trained bath aide and the untrained person the first home health care service had sent us.

For Mother's Day, Desiree sent me the book "Mom" written by Dave Isay. It is about the positive relationships mothers and their children have with each other. It was a great book for me to be reading at that time; something positive as my husband lay slowly dying a little more each day. Desiree may have been thousands of miles away in New York, but she was such a wonderful support even that far away.

People need to realize that even though you may not be close by those who need you, a phone call, a book, or some type of contact is a major way of showing your support. Don't sell it short.

The morning Vern got his first Hospice bath and massage and the bath aide was finishing up with Vern in the bedroom, the massage therapist, Beth, came and went into the bedroom where Vern was getting his bath. Derek jokingly said to Sirena and me, "It's like sending him a bunch of hookers."

Sirena responded with, "Well, what a great way to send him out. The Muslims think you get seventy-two virgins when you die. Dad can enjoy them before he dies. What a way to go!"

With the good help of Sirena, Derek, the Hospice staff, and Tata, I was improving from my surgery every day. I felt I could soon take over Vern's care and let Tata go.

On May 15th, Vern woke Derek during the night and insisted he to take him to the bathroom. As he was walking from one room to the other, he fell and hit his head, and Derek couldn't lift him. He called 911. Derek said he was frightened because Vern didn't wake up before the firefighters and rescue units got here. Once they got here, they got him back in the hospital bed, and he woke up.

The firemen told Derek they remembered being here several years before. Derek remembered that happened sixteen years before. Vern's father lived with us and we had to call them because he was complaining of not being able to breathe. They took him to the hospital. We followed, and brought him back a few hours later. I'd say those firefighters have very good memories.

The following evening Morgan was here to help Derek and Tata put Vern to bed. The next morning, he couldn't get out of bed.

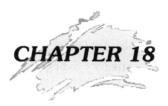

CHAPTER 18

A distant cousin, Lia Griffin, e-mailed me one day about an oscillating mattress, which is driven by a flow of air. I had never heard of this. She told me that while she was the caregiver for her grandmother, she got one. It's great for preventing bedsores as it constantly moves and shifts under the patient. I contacted Sonja Zimmer at the ALS Chapter, and she had one in her warehouse and brought it right out. It was truly a life saver, one we wished we'd known about much sooner.

One night the mattress quit working, and we had to wake Sirena's husband, Pat, to come over and help us take it off and put the hospital mattress back on. The next day, Sonja got us another one to use until she could find out what was wrong with the one we'd been using.

Each day before Derek went to work at 2:00, he would stop by and give his dad Ensure and medicine through the stomach peg. That was a big help to me.

The family room truly looked like a hospital room by that time. Oxygen tanks, electric cords for the fan to help keep Vern cool, cord for the mattress, the hospital bed, and the portable suction machine, IV pole, catheter bag, and many pillows to help cushion Vern's body to relieve the pain, pillows under his arms, under his legs, under his head, anywhere else he was hurting.

I had a cart at the end of his bed where we kept lotions, comb, hair brush, mouth swabs, baby wipes, gloves and other things that I would need quickly. We kept the extra supplies in that room, too, so that we could get them as needed.

Derek hung plastic bags on the bed so when he and I cleaned Vern up after bodily functions, they'd be handy for disposal of the used baby wipes and soiled blue pads. It was a great idea, and so helpful to have them handy.

One day, while Derek and I were cleaning him up, Vern commented, "You are doing something for me, son, that I never did for you. I never changed a diaper on any of you kids, let alone a poop job."

Derek helped me clean up many of his dad's poop jobs. Vern's legs were so heavy to pick up and move and hold in place. It truly was a two person job.

We began shutting the curtain in the family room as a signal to others that we needed privacy to take care of his poop jobs or for him to have time to truly rest. We had so much company. Even though many people only stayed a few minutes, some stayed much longer, and there was a steady stream of visitors. It wore Vern out. I finally typed a message "If the front drape is closed, Vern is resting and doesn't want to be disturbed. Thank you for understanding."

It worked. People were thoughtful, and didn't ring the doorbell when they saw the drape closed. When the Hospice social worker, Janine Carpenter, and nurse Kelly came, they thanked me for that, because they said they knew he wasn't getting enough rest because of too much commotion.

The month of May arrived, and still no wheelchair. Vern would have loved to have been able to just sit in it. On May 18th, the VA occupational therapist, who ordered the wheelchair, called to say that the wheelchair had been delivered to Fort Lewis Army Base. They wanted Vern to come down and do the last minute adjustments to fit him before we could pick it up. I told her, "He is bedridden now and can't get in the car, let alone ride from Federal Way to the base hospital to have final adjustments made"

The last we heard it was supposed to have been done in March. Here it was the middle of May and now he was unable to get out of bed.

"You get him down here and we can get him out of the car," she continued.

"He can't get out of bed," I told her again.

"What do you want me to do with it?" she asked.

I bet you know what I wanted to tell her without me spelling it out. I know it wasn't her fault, but I had called many times asking about the status of the wheelchair when he was failing so fast. I knew if it didn't come soon he'd never get to use it, and he was looking forward to being able to go around the neighborhood and visit with his friends. He missed being outside so much.

One of the reasons we had set up the hospital bed in the family room was because the large window there allowed him to see what was going on outside. But he missed actually being out there.

The medical professionals need to realize that a lot of ALS patients fail fast and need to be treated differently from those with a long term illness. It is hard to predict how long they will live. Few are long term patients.

May 18th, Vern decided to stop taking nourishment through his stomach peg. He   said he only wanted the medicine to make him comfortable. He didn't want to live like that, where he had no control over his bodily functions and I had to clean up after him. I told him I'd changed a lot of baby diapers and it didn't bother me to do these things for him. He said he had no quality of life left.

He then told me, "Once I knew I'd lose the ability to write, I wrote each of you a personal note and put it in the Trust book in a manila envelope. I don't want you to read them until after I'm gone." I honored his wish.

On May 20, 2010, my physical therapist discharged me. Vern's brother, Vic, and his wife, Ann, came the following day for a three day visit with Vern. They were so faithful in coming to give him support. It was almost a month after my surgery. It was a break for me. Ann took over cooking breakfast each day. One evening while they were here, Sirena brought dinner from the Olive Garden. Another night we had homemade chicken noodle soup that friends had brought. It was nice to only have to warm something up rather than have to cook from scratch.

Tata was a keeper. Vern loved her. She would massage him and sing to him and suction him, since he could no longer swallow. She was a real boost for him. He even let her comb his hair if she wanted to. That was a big surprise. They would laugh and talk and he looked forward to her coming each evening.

I was sitting at the table one evening, eating dinner when Tata arrived. Vern told me to give her something to eat. She said she wasn't used to our type of food she was only used to eating African food. He insisted she try what I was eating. She took two bites and didn't eat the rest. She got up from the table and went in to the family room to take care of him. After she left he told me, "You are not to eat when there are other people here."

"Then I would never eat, Vern, because there are always people here." He again instructed me not to eat in front of other people. If I hadn't had an opportunity to eat before Tata got here I would take a snack of some sort into our office and eat it in there. I lost 16 pounds during that time until he passed away, since it was almost impossible to find time to eat when no one was here.

Desiree's family called on the 21st of May, and we got on the speaker phone with them. Vern dozed off as he was talking to them. On the 22nd our oldest grandson, Dustin, and his girl friend came to visit his Papa. Vern ended up saying his goodbyes to Dustin. Dustin told him, "Hang in there because I still have a couple more final exams at college, then I'll be home."

"If I'm lucky I'll be dead. If not, I'll still be around." was Vern's response to him. Then Vern told me to give Dustin his final education payments so I didn't have to worry about it anymore. We had contributed to his college education each year. And we still had two years to go. I wrote that final check for Dustin and handed it to him.

There were many visitors that day, so it was busy here. I fed them pizza and several of them cleaned up the mess. They kept telling me to sit down, but, I knew my limitations and wouldn't do anything that I thought would undo my surgery.

During the night of May 26th Vern was dreaming I was in bed with him and he was patting me on the butt. He asked Derek, "Do you know who is in bed with me?" As Vern was smiling, Derek said, "Yes, two pillows." The next morning when they told me about this we all had a good laugh.

That evening as I lay on the sofa waiting for Derek to finish his shift at work, I told Vern, "You are an incredible man, Vern, and our kids are lucky to have you for a father. I'm really proud of you and what you have accomplished in life."

That next morning Vern told me when we were alone., "When it is quiet like this and only the two of us, it seems like there is a radio by the phone playing "Amazing Grace and Rock of Ages softly." That made us both cry, and as I was sobbing he continued, "They aren't through playing yet, Honey."

He then told me it had been going on for four days. I didn't know if he really knew the time-line or not. He was very sharp in his mind so he may have known. I should have asked the Hospice nurse when she was here that day if that had any significance.

At 3:35 p.m., he called me into the room and said, "Listen, they are now playing Glory, Glory, Hallelujah, the truth is marching on.

Do you hear it?"

I didn't hear it and replied, "They must be playing it too softly for me to hear." But, I was concerned about him hearing this music as I thought the end must be very near. He must have felt that way too, because he asked me to call Mike Webb and ask who with the Veterans Administration I should I contact at the time of his death.

A friend brought her guitar and serenaded him with western songs and a few religious songs. As she was leaving, Tata arrived. She brought her iPhone with some African music for him to listen to, and he seemed to enjoy that, too.

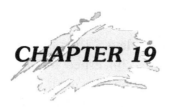

CHAPTER 19

At five o'clock on the morning of May 27th, Vern asked Derek to wake me. Derek thought he'd probably made a mess and wanted to tell me that I needed to help clean up a poop job. When I got to the side of Vern's bed, I threw back the covers, grabbed a glove and a baby wipe. He said, "It's not that! I'm dying. Call Sirena and have her come."

Derek called her, waking her from a sound sleep, "Do I have time to take my kids to school?" she asked in her groggy state.

"He says he's dying so you probably should come now." Derek answered.

That jolted her awake and she realized what was going on. She called someone to take her kids to school and rushed here from her home 25 minutes away.

I asked him, "Do you want me to call Desiree so you can talk to her?"

He answered, "No, she'll know when I fly over New York."

We all sat by his side, held his hands, talked, cried, and laughed. The whole gamut of emotions surfaced. At some point, he said he was hot and asked us to remove the sheet that was covering him. We sat there for at least an hour. Then he said, "Okay you can pull the sheet up now."

In silent communication between the two siblings, Sirena and Derek each reached down and pulled the sheet up over his head. Just like in the old western movies when some one has died.

"No, not that!" he told them. Then we all had to laugh. Often, laughter was a release from all the stress we were enduring. I'm sure that at times others felt we were being heartless, but laughter helped all of us.

A few more minutes passed and he said, "The good Lord just told me 'You can't call the shots, you aren't in charge anymore.' So I guess I'm not going to die now after all. Sorry I bothered you. Guess you can get on with your day."

On May 29th I received my sister, Alzada's, obituary in the mail along with the card handed out at her funeral services. I read it to Vern and about five minutes later he said, "Alzada never told you about all those awards, did she?"

"What awards are you talking about?" I asked.

"Jerry just came to me and told me about all the nursing awards she received because she could go into the lungs of people who were having problems like me, coughing, and she could bring up all that phlegm and save people's lives. She was known all around the world for going deeper than anyone thought possible. She won nineteen awards at the twenty hospitals she worked at." After Vern told me the story, I knew he was having hallucinations. She never worked at twenty hospitals, maybe two or three at the most.

Later, when some of our neighbors came to visit Vern told them the same thing about my sister and her awards. I couldn't tell them he was hallucinating because he was lying right there in the bed.

Memorial Day has always been a busy day for me since my oldest brother died. Vern and I have always gone to the cemeteries and decorated the grave sites of family and friends. This year, I had not been released by the surgeon to drive, so it was the first year since 1970 that I had not done it. And it looked like the next year I would be adding Vern to the list of sites I would need to visit.

Mike Webb, his wife and, the neighbor who introduced us to Mike came over to visit Vern after they had gone to Mt. Tahoma

National Cemetery. Vern really enjoyed that. We hadn't seen Mike for quite a while. When they stopped by, Mike had all the death benefit forms ready for me to file when the time came. Mike saw to it that the VA determined Vern was "housebound" so that Vern's compensation included a special monthly compensation on top of his 100 percent disability. He also asked Veterans Affairs to consider an even higher benefit due to his need for "aid and attendance." We had so much to thank him for.

We wanted to give him a gift to show our appreciation for all he did for us, and Mike said he couldn't accept any gifts. Vern insisted and Mike continued to refuse but finally said if we really wanted to do something, we could make a donation to the DAV in his name. We did that.

Vern's aunt and uncle in Reno called to see how Vern was doing. I had a hard time keeping my emotions in check. As the end grew closer, it was harder and harder.

The next day, Derek turned his dad in bed and then headed off to work. He only got a few feet down the road and he saw a transformer blow. He came back as he knew the oscillating mattress would plunge to the bed frame. There wasn't much we could do but wait for the electricity to come back on. Poor Vern was crumpled up on the deflated mattress until it was restored to the proper position of inflation.

June 1st, Vern asked me to call the Hospice chaplain to come see him. The chaplain had called several times to see if he could make a house call, and Vern always refused to have him come. I was surprised when he asked me to call him. "I'm tired of fighting this disease, and just want to pass on. I'm having trouble doing that, and I want to see if the chaplain can help me."

The chaplain came to our home and spent about an hour and a half. Nice man. Vern liked him too. I was with Vern and the chaplain most of that time, but I was having a hard time controlling my emotions so I walked out to the sunroom for about fifteen minutes, leaving them alone to talk. As the chaplain was leaving, Vern told him he could hear them singing Amazing Grace and the chaplain said, "That should be comforting to you." Vern assured him it was. Vern told me the next day, "After the chaplain's visit yesterday, I don't think about dying any more. I had a peaceful night."

Mary North, our cleaner, was dusting the book shelves in the family room one day and Vern asked her, "Do you hear the radio playing church music?"

Mary responded, "Yes, it's beautiful," even though there was no radio in that room.

Then he asked, "Would you turn up the volume?"

She answered, "Yes," and he seemed satisfied.

June 2nd, our friend, Susie, came from California for a four day visit. Susie and I met in 1954 as telephone operators in Moses Lake, Washington and have been friends ever since. She knew it was going to be the last time she was going to see Vern alive, and she wanted to let him know how much he meant to her.

In all the years we've known each other, Susie got the impression that Vern didn't believe in prayers, but something kept nagging at her as she was packing for the trip that she should bring her prayer book. The urge was so strong that she packed it in her suitcase, and after she arrived, one morning it seemed like the perfect time for her to talk to him about it. She went to his bedside with her prayer book in hand, and said, "Vern, I have something I feel is very important that I would like to do for you."

He asked her, "What would that be? I don't need anything."

"Oh, Vern, I just had to bring my old prayer book because there is one prayer in there that I want to say for you."

He responded, "Well, I would like that."

While holding his hand, she read, "O Father of mercies and God of all comfort, our only help in time of need; I humbly beseech thee to behold, visit, and relieve thy sick servant, Vern Warner, for whom my prayers are desired. Look upon Vern with the eyes of thy mercy; comfort him with a sense of thy goodness; preserve him from the temptations of the enemy; and give him patience under his ALS affliction. In thy good time, enable Vern to lead the residue of his life in thy fear, and to thy glory; and grant that finally he may dwell with thee in life everlasting; through Jesus Christ our Lord, Amen."

When she finished, Vern was crying. She asked him if he would like another prayer and he said, "Oh, yes, Susie, I need another one." While continuing to hold his hand she said another prayer for him and when she finished he told her, "Thank you so much for those prayers, I already feel different!" Then they both cried.

Our son-in-law, Gene, sent Vern a very emotional letter stating that he admired how Vern's "bright spirit and amazing resilient sense of humor come powerfully through despite your illness. You have set the bar high."

It was only one of many comments about the wonderful example Vern set as to how to act when faced with great adversity. An email from my friend, Marjorie, states, "Delores, I hope you know what an inspiration you and Vern are to me, and no doubt many others who will walk this way. You are laying down a path through the darkest of dark valleys, showing us how to keep on going forward toward the new and very difficult day that lies at the end of the road. I am amazed by your deep, sweet, unswerving love for one another, your ability to touch and talk together even through this long, hard, sad time."

These and other messages gave us more courage to face what we had to, when at times it was frightening and overwhelming.

I have always taken pride in my yard and flower beds, but I had no time for them that year. In June, Sirena, Morgan and Erika weeded and planted the flower beds with impatiens, mowed the front pasture and the lawns. And they brushed the horses. It always lifted my spirits just to look out the windows and see that it was done.

My ironing had also been neglected. When Susie was here she ironed every last piece that hung in the laundry room. She had just had heart surgery six weeks before I had my surgery. I kept begging her to stop but she wouldn't until it was all in the closets. What a relief that was, to see it out of the laundry room.

Another friend had come to visit Vern again, and Tata was in the room taking care of him. As the friend was bidding Vern goodbye, she leaned over and kissed him. Vern said Tata got the funniest look on her face. After the friend left the room, Tata told Vern, "In Africa if a woman kissed another woman's husband she'd be dead."

Vern explained to her that in America it is just a sweet gesture. She restated, "In Africa she be dead."

When he told me that, I said, "If that was true here there would be a lot of dead women that have come to see you."

Vern said to Derek and me, "I want to dangle my feet over the edge of the bed. Do you two think you can hold me in that position?" Derek and I got him upright. It was the first time since he'd been bedridden that he got to sit up. I massaged his back, brushed and combed his hair.

He said, "That felt so good, maybe I CAN sit in my wheelchair." Then he asked us to start giving him Ensure and water again. Once we did that, much to our astonishment, he perked up, and his catheter bag showed his urine turning from the color of Bock beer to the color of Bud Light.

June 8th, Vern started off having a bad day. He was hallucinating a lot, rambling on something about Filipino women making him tea, and asking if he'd eaten yet, wanting to know what he'd had for breakfast. That type of thing. I don't think he had a rational moment all day. One time when he spoke I didn't understand him so I leaned closer and asked him what he wanted, and he opened his eyes, which were glassy and answered, "I'm not talking to you."

Early evening he seemed to have some rational moments. He asked for coffee so I gave him some. We put his liquids in the bag on the IV pole which had a tube attached to it that we placed in his stomach peg. He wanted his hair combed again. Then he told me to take care of the bookwork. He always worried about that getting done. I felt I had enough to worry about without trying to keep his bookwork up to date. I hadn't even gone grocery shopping since before my surgery which was seven weeks earlier.

A new sleeping pill was ordered for him. We hoped he wouldn't have so many hallucinations. They were sometimes funny. He would say, "Make sure there is enough food. Make sure you have something everyone will like." "Do you have the food ready?" One time he said, "The people are going to be really surprised," I asked him why they were going to be surprised, and he said, "Because Tata is serving the African food." And he smiled.

One of my best memories of this time was photographing Vern with some of the Hospice staff. He loved the attention. I got pictures of Janine, Kelly, the bath aide, Tena. and massage therapist, Beth, with him lying in the hospital bed. Later I also got pictures of him with Tata.

It was time for my six weeks check up after my surgery. I had gone home in one of the hospital gowns since no one told me I might have a catheter bag, which meant the slacks I had worn to the hospital before surgery weren't going to work. Now, I wanted to return the hospital gown, so I washed and ironed it. I also wanted to thank the hospital staff for the care they'd given me. Since the doctor's office was near the hospital, I combined the two stops.

At my request, Sirena had picked up a large box of doughnuts, and some Life Savers for me to leave at the nurses' station at the hospital. I'd already had Derek pick up a box of See's candy for them.

For some reason, I was put in the maternity section of the hospital. When we got to the door to give them the thank you package, Sirena rang the bell so they could let us in. The nurse who answered the bell asked, "Can I help you?"

Sirena, my little RN announced, "I have a delivery." All the nurses thought that was pretty funny (so did I) considering the area we were in.

I had the See's candy, the hospital gown and life savers all in a gift bag and Sirena carried the box of doughnuts. I told them that the doughnuts were for the certified nursing assistant who had provided me with the "donut" at the hospital because my bottom was so sore it hurt to sit. Even after six weeks those groin muscles, which the nurses jokingly called, "yes and no" muscles, were very sore and I was still using the donut at home. I had unexpected incisions there. Vern told me next time I have surgery to find a doctor that had smaller hands. Later I found out that one of the nurses at the station, who hadn't been assigned to me, was a good friend of Sirena's. She had come in to my room one day to give me a pep talk when I was so sick and vomiting.

The nurses loved the gifts, and that made my day. They were so good to me at the hospital, each and every one of them.

I was in the office doing some paperwork when Derek entered and said, "Dad wants his left elbow rubbed."

As I was massaging his elbow he passed gas and I kind of chuckled, and Vern said, "You laugh but the old Indian chief has always told me it's a special elbow." He repeated that three times. Who was I to argue with an old Indian chief? So I continued to pacify him by rubbing his elbow.

June 11th, as I was crushing his medication in order to put it through his stomach peg he called my name. When he was rational he would tell me when his meds were due and which ones, although I didn't need him telling me as I had made a list of what was due when. He constantly called me every five minutes. I couldn't be out of his sight. Even when Tata was there and I was supposed to be resting, he kept calling me. This time, he didn't give me a chance to finish preparing the medication and yelled at me again. I answered, "What?"

When I walked into the room Tata said to him, "You call her too much. When I first come here to work and you call her she answer, 'Yes, Honey.' now she say 'What?' When I'm here you call me not her. That's why I'm here."

Vern told me to give Tata a bonus of $50.00 so she could go to a Red Lobster Restaurant. They had watched a commercial on TV about the restaurant, and he asked her if she had ever been to one. When she said no he told me to give her the bonus so she could take her aunt as well. Later she told him they enjoyed their meal.

That evening Sirena and Pat were here and Vern decided he wanted to "walk" to his lift chair. Of course he couldn't walk. It took Pat, Tata, Sirena, Dustin and Derek to get him to his lift chair. He stayed there about an hour before going back to bed. He then determined he was going to sit in his wheelchair when it was to be delivered on June 17th.

The following day I was able to take care of him by myself while Derek did work outside that needed to be done. I started hurting again, in the area where my hernia had been. I decided I had to be more careful about straining myself as I worked with Vern.

Vern changed his mind about the wheelchair, and he had me call the VA hospital and tell them NOT to bring it, and to cancel that appointment which they said would be a three hour ordeal. It was the first time in VA history that they were going to deliver a wheelchair to a home, but our social worker had raised enough hell about him not being able to go to the base hospital that they'd agreed to deliver it.

Even though they were bringing it to our home, Vern told me he was just too weak to be jostled around, and he didn't think he'd even be able to use it. I talked to nurse Kelly, and she agreed with that decision. I then called and left a message canceling the delivery.

The next day there was a knock at the door, and I was surprised to see the VA staff standing there. I asked them to come in and told them I had called and canceled. They said they hadn't picked up their messages from the day before. I asked them to go visit with Vern.

They left his room and could see he couldn't move, and we went to the sunroom. I told them, "As you can see he will never be able to use the chair. You can take it back and give it to someone else. That's what I have been so concerned about, that it would come too late for him to be able to use it. It has taken far too long." I was angry but I was civil to them even though they had promised it would arrive much earlier, when Vern could still use his hands.

Later, Derek reminded me that Vern was the first ALS patient they had dealt with and that I needed to realize they didn't know or understand the urgency in getting things done quickly when dealing with ALS patients. He was right. It was obvious from their expressions, they never expected to find him in that condition, even though I had told her he was bed-bound. He was really out of it, and couldn't even properly visit with them.

Vern told me earlier in the day, "If I have to continue with a week like I just had, I don't want to live ." We had hoped that the wheelchair would give him the incentive to go on. But, it was too late getting here.

Again I told them to take it back and give it to someone else. One of them said, "Well, when he rallies maybe he can use it."

"He has ALS he isn't going to rally." I said.

They then decided they'd leave it anyway, saying that when he was done with it they'd come back and pick it up if I wanted to return it to them at that time. It was Vern's chair, they explained, and he could do whatever he wanted with it. Then they left. "I'd like to see a picture of the wheelchair, honey, if you would take one and show me." Vern said after they left.

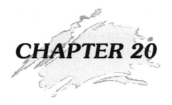

CHAPTER 20

"I've been thinking about giving Tata another bonus once her work here is done. Is that okay with you?" I asked Vern.

"Yes, if that is what you want to do." he answered.

"How much do you think I should give her?" We discussed it briefly and we both had the same figure in mind.

June 18th, Vern asked me to call Janine, the Hospice social worker, because he was tired of fighting the disease. I caught her at the office. She'd just been out in the field and was starting on her paperwork. She dropped it and came right over. She discussed his fight with ALS with him, his emotional feelings, and his options. He had told her he just wanted something to let him sleep, no food, nothing to drink, just something to let him be comfortable.

She called Nurse Kelly, and she too dropped everything and rushed over. Nurse Kelly had called the head Hospice doctor before coming and now she discussed Vern's options with him. Vern was adamant that he couldn't fight the disease any more. She told him about all the things available to him if he chose to continue fighting. He rejected them all. He didn't want to live like that.

After having an open discussion about everything, Vern said again he was exhausted and had no quality of life, and no muscle control. He was paralyzed and could only move his eyes and talk. It was getting more and more difficult for him to breathe, which caused him a great deal of anxiety. He again asked for medication to relax him, ease his breathing, and make him more comfortable. Right along, he'd made it clear to all of us that he wanted no extreme measures taken to prolong his death. What he asked for was simply a measure of comfort while nature took it's course. We all agreed on medication to maximize his comfort, reduce his pain, and calm his restless sleep. He said, "This is no way to live."

They asked me how I felt about that. I said I would honor his wishes, as I could see what he was going through and I would want the same thing if it were me. Boy! That was a hard thing to say. Vern and I went back a long ways. I met him when I was 16 and we married two years later, so he was a huge part of my life for 59 years. I really knew no other life without him. Now, I had to say I honored his decision to die. That was very difficult.

As we were leaving the room I asked Janine and Kelly, "Well, if he is going to be sleeping then I don't need to pay Tata to come back, do I?"

They said it was up to me, but Vern heard what I'd said, and he spoke loudly, "I want to die knowing Tata is massaging my body, I want her here until I'm gone." That was June 18th.

Tata had never missed coming a single day after she started working for us. She never took a day off. She was so reliable, always on time, neat, and always ready to get to work. Vern told me he could relax so much easier with her massaging his body. It seemed to help relieve some of the pain and muscles aches. I said, "Okay." And I kept her coming each evening as she had been doing.

I was the one who gave him the first pill that would sedate him. I crushed it along with the other medications he was taking. I sat at the breakfast bar that I had set up as a lab center for us to work with his meds, with tears rolling down my cheeks, knowing that this was truly the beginning of the end and I was the one who was administering it to him. Not an easy job to undertake even though it was what he wanted.

Usually when a patient makes the decision to be sedated, they go to Hospice House, where a doctor monitors the patient. Vern refused to go, even as he insisted on being sedated. The Hospice staff said since Sirena was an RN, and I had worked in a doctor's office for years, and our house was very clean and orderly, and we had taken such wonderful care of him so far, they would allow us to sedate him at home.

Derek became an expert at giving him his medication in the stomach peg. He had it down pat, how to keep it from getting all over Vern and the bedding. He always gave Vern his dose right before going to his swing shift job.

June 21st, the third day of being sedated, Vern was doing a lot of talking in his sleep. Some of what he says I could understand, other things I couldn't. One time he said, "The pictures are horrible, get rid of the pictures, they are terrible."

I was standing by his bed massaging his arms, and replied, "Okay, I will get rid of them."

He was agitated and a few minutes later he yelled, "Get rid of the pictures, you didn't get rid of the pictures, I don't like the pictures." I didn't know what to say. I know a sedated patient can hear someone talking to them, but he was so upset, I didn't know how to put him at ease.

Another time he kept calling my name. Sirena was here and we were both by his bedside. She told me, "Mom, tell him you are okay and that you are right here." I did that and he calmed down.

He kept talking about the holidays: Thanksgiving, Christmas and Easter dinner, always asking me if I had it ready or if I had enough food for everyone." It was like he was obsessed with food. He was always the perfect host, making sure everyone was fed, and there was something everyone liked.

When Janine and Kelly came that day I told them of his ramblings and hallucinations. I thought it was the medication. They explained to me it was his process of passing. They said he was reviewing his life like a movie. They said some people do it in a few hours, some take days. And, when he was saying "Take the pictures away", it was because he was reliving something in his life he'd done that he didn't like and didn't want to review. They said "We've all done things in our lives we wished we hadn't, and in the process of dying we will review all those things."

I told them, "I thought your heart had to stop beating and you actually died before you reviewed your life. I thought you had actually passed away before that happened." They told me I was witnessing someone reviewing his life in the process of dying. That was an education for me.

As I was sitting by the side of his bed late one night, holding his hand, waiting for Derek to come relieve me so I could go to bed, Vern asked, "Who are all these people and what are they doing here" After what Janine and Kelly told me, I knew that the end was very near.

The morning of June 22nnd, Vern said, "Susie", and Derek said "What?", and he said , "I'm talking to Susie."

My note in my journal that evening reads: "Last evening as Tata was massaging Vern's neck she leaned close to his ear and asked him, 'Do you know who is massaging you?' and he slowly opened his eyes, which he hadn't done for the past few days and said, 'Yes, Tata.' He never spoke again.

She had told me when she first came that evening that she had a dream about the two of them the night before. They were walking down a street. She said he was in his hospital gown and they were laughing and just having a great time, and people were staring at them but they didn't care because they were having so much fun. Then her dream switched to me welcoming her in the door to tell her he had passed away.

I was still having problems with my surgical site and had put off going to the doctor because my time was so limited. But, Vern and Derek had insisted a couple weeks before that I make an appointment with the doctor and Derek would stay with Vern if I could get it done before he had to go to work.

I wanted to see my primary physician rather than my surgeon. But it turned out I had to make an appointment with the doctor that shares her office, because June 23rd was my doctor's day off. I had an 11:00 a.m. appointment.

Suddenly at five minutes to 11:00 as I was sitting in the waiting room I started crying. I couldn't stop crying. I wiped the tears away. Two gentlemen who were also waiting kept looking at me. I was embarrassed because I didn't know what had brought the tears on. But, I had the feeling I had to get home. I was just about to stand and leave when the nurse's assistant called me back.

I had never met this doctor before. As I waited for her to come in, I kept telling myself to control myself. By the time she came in, I wasn't sobbing any more. I told her about my problem, she checked me out, and told me to go back to the surgeon. As she started out the door I started sobbing again and she stepped back in the room and said, "Are you okay?"

"My husband has ALS and I don't know how much longer I'm going to have him," I answered.

"Are you okay to drive?" she asked me.

"Yes, I have to get home." I hurried and dressed, got in the car, and drove home.

I knew the bath aide, Tena, was supposed to give Vern a bath at the time I'd be gone. When I drove in the driveway I saw a different car than what Tena usually drove. Derek was sitting in the living room and a different bath aide was giving Vern his bath in the family room. Derek asked me what the doctor said, but I felt this urgency to go see Vern. Still, since I had not seen this bath aide before, I didn't want to disturb her while she was bathing him. I didn't know if she'd like my intruding while she was doing her job. As I was telling Derek what the doctor said, the bath aide hollered for us to come quick.

"He's passing." she said as we entered the room. I hadn't been home 10 minutes. Derek and I stood by his bed. I touched his chest where his heart was barely beating, and then I touched the carotid artery in his neck, and kept my hand there until the last faint heart beat. He was gone. His suffering had come to an end. The bath aide reached over and closed his eyes. I leaned over and kissed him on the forehead. Then the flood of tears came. He had faced this disease with courage, strength, grace and dignity. He had finished one journey and was on to a new one.

Nurse Kelly happened to be ten minutes early for her appointment with us. What a blessing that was. She arrived just two or three minutes after he passed away. It was Sirena's day off, so Derek called her at home and she rushed over. Kelly took over calling the funeral home, and taking care of all the things that the family is too upset to do.

When the neighbors and friends found out Vern had passed away they came to our home with their condolences. When Tata came to take care of him, I welcomed her at the door and slipped a thank you card and the bonus Vern and I had agreed on into her pocket. When she entered our home and saw all the people there she said, "He's gone, isn't he?" Just like in her dream. I confirmed that, and invited her to sit down.

She joined some of us at the table. I was sitting beside her and she asked, "Do you have a picture of him that I can have?" I went to our home office and took a picture of him that I had on the wall and gave it to her. It was a portrait shot I'd taken of him a few years before, one of my favorites. The tears fell down her cheeks as she looked at that handsome face.

Later when I talked to Desiree she said that 11:00 our time she had the feeling he was passing.

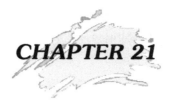

CHAPTER 21

I contacted the VA to come pick up the unused wheelchair. They gave it to another ALS patient that was on their list of those needing one just like it.

When I started getting my information ready for the IRS my friend, Susie, called me and told me to make sure I claimed the wheelchair as a deduction because it was made for Vern and was his to do with as he wanted. The VA had told him that at the time he was measured for it, and he asked what we were to do with it once he passed away. I called the VA hospital and asked for a value of the wheelchair so I could claim it as a donation. They wouldn't tell me. They said I couldn't claim it as a donation even though it had never been used. Susie insisted it was okay and to call the IRS.

The person at the IRS said, "Yes, you can claim it as a donation, but you have to get a written statement from the VA saying you donated it, the date of the contribution, and the value of the chair. You will only get a portion of the value as a donation but you can do that." The VA refused to give me a receipt documenting I'd donated it back to them.

Please be aware, if you donate a wheelchair to an organization rather than a private party you can claim it on your income tax report. I didn't get to claim it because of lack of co-operation from the VA hospital at Fort Lewis. We had made many monetary donations to organizations that helped us, and we also donated several things to the ALS warehouse, such as his lift chair, bedding, the new chrome grab bars that we never installed in the shower, the bath bench, water proof mattress pad cover, and so on. All those things I was able to deduct.

I put Vern's obituary in the Seattle Times, the Wenatchee paper and the Grand Coulee paper (where he was raised), but when I checked how much it would cost for our local paper, they told me it would be at least $600. I told them I would use that money for food at the reception. The Grand Coulee paper printed it for free.

While I was planning the reception for his funeral services and the menu, Derek kept saying I should plan for a hundred people. I kept telling him there weren't going to be that many people there. He said, "Trust me, Mom, there are going to be a lot of people there." Then he added, "Mom, you know Dad would be saying, 'Make sure there is enough food.'" It turned out that although Derek was right about the number of people, we did have plenty of food and sent a lot of food home with others after the reception. Vern would have liked that.

I was stunned at how many people attended the services. One hundred and four people signed the guest book and we knew of at least twenty-six people that had to get back to work and didn't attend the reception where we had the guest book. All three traffic lanes were filled with cars clear out to the road. We thought they must have been there for another service, but the volunteers at the cemetery said they were all there for Vern.

About 2 weeks after Vern passed, Sirena and Derek were here helping me with paperwork. As I was looking for something in his desk, it suddenly hit me he told me had written each of us a note while he could still write. I told Sirena and Derek, and I looked in the Trust book where Vern had told me he put the notes, but they weren't there. We looked everywhere we could think of that he may have put them, but we couldn't find a manila envelope with his notes. The following day Derek went to the safe and found them.

Sirena says it is one of the most treasured gifts he had ever given her. He had attached, or included, things that we had given him over the years in each individual envelope. They were also things I never knew he'd saved in his desk. But, then, I never looked in his desk. Now when I did, I found many cards I'd given him over the years, Valentines, Father's Day cards, birthday cards, and Christmas cards, that I had signed with sentimental comments at the bottom.

Eighteen months passed between the day Vern's diagnosis of ALS was confirmed and the day of his passing. They were days filled with struggles, tears, difficulties, and pain. But as I look back on those months of Vern's illness and his passing, I can see much more clearly that in spite of the occasional, and clearly understandable, bad temperament of a dying man, and my own sheer exhaustion, I learned to weather the bad times, and enjoy the good moments of companionship and our shared humor.

Vern and I switched roles. In the past, I was the one who was always dependent on him, he became completely dependent on me. He had always been the provider, and then I became the provider for his every need. Suddenly all of the responsibilities fell on my shoulders and I managed, somehow, to stand up to the test. I accompanied Vern on his last journey here on earth, as he slipped away to face a new journey without me. It was a time when, hard as it was, I truly came to understand the vow I took when we were married: "In sickness and health, 'till death do us part."

CHAPTER 22

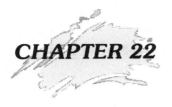

I would like to share the note that Vern wrote to me with you now.

My Darling Wife
4-02-2009

First off thank you for being my wife. You have always been there for me and made me feel that I could succeed at whatever. You gave me 3 wonderful children that I'm proud of, you were a great and loving mother, you were a loving and giving wife and always gave ahead of your own wants or needs.

I'm not a good writer but want you to know I've always been proud to have you as my wife and want you to know I'm so sorry for putting you through this now, and I want you to go on after I'm gone and enjoy what's left of your life and I'll be waiting for you later after you fulfill your life but don't hurry. I'll wait.

I love you so much
Vern

Why did he find it hard to tell me this when he was alive? Why did he tell me to wait until he'd died before I read this note?

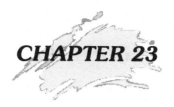

CHAPTER 23

IMPORTANT THINGS TO REMEMBER

Veterans Affairs

If you are a veteran: The Veterans Affairs have accepted responsibility for veterans with ALS. But, you MUST contact a DAV (Disabled American Veteran) representative or a PAV (Paralyzed Veterans Administration) representative. Mike Webb was invaluable to us in helping fill out paperwork and insisted that the VA expedite claims because of Vern's age and the disease.

Hospice

While talking with Kelly Chumbley and Janine Carpenter (of Hospice) they stated, they encourage patients and families to open the door to talking with their doctor about what lies ahead, when a cure is not an option. A decision facilitated by the doctor will be made as to when Hospice should be contacted. They will evaluate the patient and make a decision as to when their help is needed. They said it is important to get the paperwork done early so they can have it on file and ready to go when one needs them. Doctors are becoming more comfortable discussing end of life issues with their patients, but sometimes it is still families who have to advocate for the discussion, they told me.

I didn't realize this and I waited too long. I thought I could do things myself and ended up with a five and a half hour surgery because I didn't ask for help earlier. I had dislodged my internal organs by wrestling Vern around, picking him up as he gradually lost strength and was unable to help me help him. ALS patients eventually become "dead weight" when they can no longer use their own muscles.

Hospice can provide bath aides, massage therapists, registered nurses, and social workers, all of whom are a tremendous help. We had a wonderful team assigned to us.

We always thought Hospice workers only came during the last six months of the patient's life, but that isn't true, they will come much earlier if you need help. We only had them Vern's last six weeks of life. I wish I'd contacted them earlier.

Home Health Care Agencies & Housekeeping Service

We didn't have very good luck with the first home health care agency we contacted but the second one was a winner. Hospice Social Workers have a list that you can choose from. The first agency we contacted was from a recommendation of a good friend but we didn't get the same person that was assigned to her father. Don't be afraid to let them go if you aren't satisfied with them. Get another agency. There are a lot of them out there.

My husband and I were pretty particular about our home being clean, and I couldn't have kept it up the way we liked if it hadn't been for a housekeeping service. We were fortunate enough to be able to afford one. If you can afford it I highly recommend it.

If you are going to take care of the patient at home, I find it to be a necessity.

Choose Clothing That Is Easy To Put On the Patient

As the patient's muscles deteriorate they become harder to dress. Imagine dressing an infant, one that can't help you put their arms or legs in their clothing. Toward the end, I purchased nice pajamas from Nordstrom Rack when I could no longer put Vern's jeans on him. I pressed them and had him looking sharp for the many visitors that he had. Neither of us was ashamed as he sat in his nice pajamas, yet they made it easy for me to dress him.

Lift Chair

When the patient has difficulty getting up out of a chair, you can purchase a lift chair that has controls to lift the patient into a standing position. This is really helpful to both caregiver and patient. It gives the patient that last little bit of independence to stand without having to ask for help.

Bidet

This was a tremendous suggestion from the ALS patient services director of our local ALS chapter, Sonja Zimmer. When the patient becomes unable to wipe themselves after a bathroom visit, they are able to use the remote control that comes with the bidet. When my husband could no longer control his fingers (after accidentally hitting the enema button) I would take the remote control into the hallway, and when he'd finished he would tell me and I'd hit the posterior button to wash him off. It was especially nice when he had diarrhea. We purchased a portable bidet, and they make them to fit on any type of toilet.

Speaker Phone

Once Vern couldn't hold the phone in his hands, one of us had to hold it to his ear, which was uncomfortable for him as well as us. We purchased a speaker phone, and it was a true blessing. He could talk as long as he wanted and it wasn't uncomfortable for any of us.

Transport Chair and Wheelchair

We purchased a transport chair first. Transport chairs are those chairs with wheels that you sometimes see people pushing like a wheelchair, only they are lighter weight and can be folded and put in a vehicle. You can use them when the patient finds it exhausting to walk very far.

You need to put an order in for a wheelchair months in advance of needing one. They are custom made to the patient and it takes forever to get them made.

Massaging & Cradles for Hands

The patient loves to be massaged. It is relaxing to them and helps alleviate the pain somewhat. It helps to reduce the swelling of the hands. The cradles that go under the forearm and hands helps keep the hands from curling painfully.. The massaging just feels good.

Terry Cloth Bathrobe

I was having trouble getting Vern dry after a shower, before he became too tired to keep standing. An occupational therapist suggested I try putting a terry cloth bathrobe on him as soon as I got him out of the shower, and then have him lie on the bed while I dried his legs, feet and toes. Then when I pulled him up into a sitting position the rest of his body was dry from the bathrobe. That worked wonders.

Baby Wipes & Blue Pads

While Vern was still able to wipe himself after going to the bathroom I purchased baby wipes because they were easier for him to use before we bought the bidet.

Once he was bed-ridden, baby wipes were a life saver for me to use when I cleaned him up. The blue pads were provided to us by Hospice, and I put them under him in case of an accident or a spill-over from cleaning him up after a bowel movement. Don't be without these items.

My son put a plastic bag on the IV pole near the hospital bed we had Vern in, so it was fast and easy to dispose of these soiled items.

Stomach Peg

This is something that should be surgically done while the patient still has good lung and breathing capacity, because they are put under general anesthesia. Many patients debate about having it done including my husband, but once he decided to have it done it was easier for me to feed him. If the patient is still capable of swallowing that is fine, you don't have to use the stomach peg even if it has been surgically inserted. But when the patient can no longer swallow, you can feed him and administer his medication through the stomach peg.

It is very important for those who have pain to get pain medication, as there comes a time when they cannot swallow it. You have to keep the patient comfortable and as free from pain as possible. Not all ALS patients suffer pain, but Vern happened to be one who was in constant pain. The pain level varies from patient to patient.

Hospital Bed

We were told by the physical therapist, occupational therapist, and Vern's primary physician, that he needed a hospital bed long before the Veterans Affairs ever got him one. The government is very slow, and even though our DAV rep asked them to expedite things for him, it didn't always happen. Don't be afraid to keep asking for the bed, because the patient is much more comfortable in those beds that can be raised and lowered for them. Hospital gowns make it easier to administer medication and do the clean up jobs.

If you are not a veteran and in need of a hospital bed, Medicare will cover it, if your doctor prescribes one. You can check the Internet for more information as to where you can get one.

An Oscillating Mattress

We borrowed an oscillating mattress from the Evergreen ALS chapter. This is a mattress that has massage type rollers in it, and is run by electricity. It takes the pressure off of any one body part, so it prevents bedsores. Marvelous invention. Too expensive to buy, but we were lucky to be able to borrow that one. Vern never got a bedsore.

BiPap - breathing mask

This helps pump oxygen to the patient when he is having difficulty breathing on his own.

Suction Machine & Swabs

Keeping secretions out of the patient's mouth is important, and the suction machine helps with this. Hospice furnished us with disposable swabs to help keep his mouth clear of secretions. They also gave us a cream to put on his lips to keep them soft.

Fans

The patient's body temperature fluctuates, and when they get too warm they need to have portable fans available to keep them cool.

My Signal for Privacy

When Vern wanted to rest or needed privacy for clean-up, I closed the drape. I made a sign and placed it on the screen door, and left it there. I stated that when they saw the family room drape closed (that is where I had my husband) they knew he wanted to rest and not be disturbed, and I thanked them for understanding. That was my signal for them not to ring the doorbell or come in. It worked well. The Hospice staff was so happy I did that when they saw it, because they said he was not getting enough rest. He had too much company.

Baby Monitor

If the patient is in another room, some caregivers use a baby monitor so they can hear the patient call them, or to monitor breathing.

Veteran's Affairs Caregiver Support

Veteran's Affairs now has a caregiver support web site and phone number for those needing help. Since they didn't have that when Vern was ill, I can't give you any first hand experience with that, but want to pass on the web site and phone number to you.

The web site is http:// www.caregiver.va.gov/ and the phone number is 1-855-260-3274.

Dr. Baughter & Dr. Sims Book

Dr. Bob Baugher and Dr. Darcie Sims have a book, In The Midst of Caregiving, that is a wonderful book for caregivers to read. You can order the book by emailing Dr. Baugher at: b_kbaugher@ yahoo.com or calling him at: 425-226-2350. Cost of the book is $12.00. He also has books for sale on Amazon.com.

Websites

There is a website Lotsa Helping Hands that is helpful to some caregivers. You can announce your needs in help, and others can sign up to be available to help those in need.

I found information on the Internet at http://www.alsa.org, http://www.ncbI.nlm.nih.gov. These websites provided the statistics cited in the introduction also. I signed up for the email newsletters from our Evergreen Chapter of ALS, to get updated information. If you have a chapter near you, I highly suggest you contact them.

Epilouge

As the funeral home staff rolled Vern down the ramp to the hearse I told Sirena, "Well, he finally got to use that damn wheelchair ramp."

Sirena added, "And even on wheels." We looked at each other and she added, "Dad would be laughing at us now."

A year after Vern passed away, I received a letter from the VA asking about the cost of the remodel of one of our bathrooms that we had considered having done so I could bathe him more easily. When the contractor told us it would take him six month to complete with permits and so forth, we declined having it done. Vern said, "I'll be dead before six months is up and I don't want the house torn up for six months while I'm dying." And, indeed, he did pass away before those six months were up.

When I received that letter asking about the bathroom remodel, I wrote a note to the author of the letter stating we hadn't done the remodel. I also told her how frustrated I was that we had never been reimbursed for the wheelchair ramp. We felt we had been so fair in only asking for the cost of the materials.

I subsequently got a call from the lady to whom I'd written. "Do you still have the receipts for the wheelchair ramp?" she asked.

I answered, "I don't know if I've thrown them away or not, but I know right where to find them if I still have them."

"If you find them, send them to me," she said. "You must have talked to someone at the hospital about the reimbursement, didn't you?"

"Yes, because that was who we were told to give the receipts to." I answered.

She informed me, "Don't listen to those people at the hospital.

They don't know what is going on in our department. You need to contact us at Specially Adapted Housing, and ask for a grant or reimbursement."

I found the receipts. A couple of them were too faded to read. I sent the readable ones to her. She called when she received them. She said she would give them to her supervisor and try to get me a check for the amount of the receipts.

A few weeks later she called again, "I'm sending your reimbursement in the overnight mail." It was something I never thought I'd ever receive. Vern would have been very happy had he been alive.

In Vern's final note to me he said, "After I'm gone, enjoy what is left of your life." One late afternoon after I fed the animals and had filled a wheelbarrow with wood for the wood stove, I was trudging through the snow, pushing the wheelbarrow when tears started falling, for seemingly no particular reason. I stopped, looked up at the sky, tears still streaming down my face, and said, "Vern, is this what you meant about me enjoying my life?" it made me wonder if I was ever going to have a life after his death.

One of my friends, after losing her husband, said to me, "I just want to die and be with him, and I look forward to it." I couldn't understand how she could feel that way at the time. After Vern died, I admit there were a few days I felt the same way. Being with Vern was the only life I really knew. My life had been centered on him and now my life felt empty.

Those of us that were left behind still needed support, emotional as well as physical, but many people disappear once the patient passes on. Yes, this was a tragedy for Vern, but also for all of us who cared for him, helping him through this ordeal.

I kept hearing from others that the first year is the hardest, especially getting through holidays and special occasions. And it truly was for me. But when Thanksgiving, Christmas, and Easter rolled around, I invited family and friends for dinner. That made it much easier.

Valentine's Day was the hardest holiday for me as it has always been one of my favorites. Vern gave me my first box of chocolates on a Valentine's Day when we were dating. I loved decorating our home, picking out that special card and surprising him with a special gift. For me, the day seemed even more special than our anniversaries, and once I got past that first Valentine's Day without Vern, I knew I'd be okay.

Our anniversary came shortly after that first Valentine's Day without him. I took flowers to the cemetery, but that didn't seem as hard to get through as Valentine's Day had been.

As the days passed, I reminded myself that I still had three beautiful children and seven beautiful grandchildren to enjoy. I had friends, some of whom had gone through the same thing I was going through. My life wasn't over. Still it was a year before I decided to do something about getting on with my new life without Vern.

I saw an ad in the newspaper about the Community Center offering ballroom dance classes; something I'd always wanted to do. I talked to my granddaughter, Erika, and we decided to do it together. After the first class I talked another granddaughter, Morgan, into doing the waltz class and foxtrot class with us. Erika decided she wanted to also attend the salsa class. Next, I signed my grandson, Nathaniel, up for salsa as well as the foxtrot class. We had a blast. I loved introducing my grandkids to ballroom dancing.

My friend, Mary, had told me shortly after Vern's death, I basically knew no other life than with Vern, and now I had to adjust to him being gone and start a different life.

What once seemed normal to me has changed since Vern's

passing. I'm now accepting the new "normal". I'm living with peace, and the new normal is good. Yes, my life is different now, but I'm doing okay.

About the Author

In addition to being a wife and mother of three grown children, Delores worked in doctors' offices as a "floater" for nine years; worked as a medical assistant, lab technician, developed xrays, worked as the office manager, when the regular one was on vacation, and spent three years as a medical transcriptionist.

She is also a certified handwriting analyst who has done personnel consultation and individual personal analysis on issues of compatibility in business, marriage, friendships, and other relationships, including troubled juveniles and their families. She has worked with police departments and has lectured extensively, including educational presentations aboard cruise ships.

Delores continues to live in the house her husband built from her design, although she no longer has a mini-farm; only one peacock, some chickens and a goat roam the pastures at her residence.

Her relationship with her children and grandchildren is very close.

Ordering information:
Don't Buy Too Many Green Bananas:
Living With ALS

Price: $10.00 (U.S. funds) per copy
Add $2.00 postage for each copy

Six or more copies:
   10% Discount and free postage for U.S. orders.

Canadian and out of U.S. orders will be billed
according to postal rates.

Washington State residents add 8.9% sales tax
Please allow 2-4 weeks for delivery

To order, email Delores Warner at
greenbananas623@gmail.com
or
order on Amazon.com

Made in the USA
Middletown, DE
10 December 2019